PRAISE FOR

Adventures for Your Soul

"Shannon offers easy-to-absorb advice to help you become your happiest, most loved, highest-potential self—and best of all she makes it a fun process—my kind of gal."
—Karen Salmansohn, bestselling author of *How to Be Happy, Dammit: A Cynic's Guide to Spiritual Happiness*

"[A] profound book and a must-read for anyone that prioritizes happiness . . . This is the playbook for making small changes and shifts that will yield you large results in your happiness."
—Kristine Carlson, *New York Times* bestselling author of *Don't Sweat the Small Stuff for Women and Moms*

"Shannon Kaiser is an incredible woman on a mission to help people find peace, happiness and fulfillment in their lives. Her desire to serve others shines through all of her work."
—Gabrielle Bernstein, *New York Times* bestselling author of *May Cause Miracles*

"Shannon shares her story of vulnerability and victory and emerges as a radiant example of what is possible with a mental makeover. *Adventures for Your Soul* gives you an easy-to-follow roadmap to lasting happiness, joy, and inner transformation. People say happiness is an inside job—this is the ultimate how-to manual."
—Amy Leigh Mercree, author of *The Spiritual Girl's Guide to Dating*

continued . . .

"For many of us, feeling excited and fulfilled on a day-to-day basis can seem impossible. If you are in search of lasting happiness, then let this truly remarkable woman guide you. She reminds us all that life is supposed to be exciting, fun, and fulfilling."

—*IDEAL Magazine*

"She not only believes in the message of happiness, she lives it and breathes it. Every time I talk to Shannon, happiness finds a way in. Pick up this book and breathe in some happiness into your heart and mind."

—Christine Arylo, self-love author of *Madly in Love with ME, the Daring Adventure of Becoming Your Own Best Friend*

"Shannon shines a fresh light and adds much needed beauty to us all. Her positivity is infectious and *Adventures for Your Soul* helps readers banish the Big Fat Lies of their Inner Critic and Inner Mean Girl and turn towards the truth of their Inner Wisdom. I highly recommend it for anyone who is ready to experience more happiness and everyday joy."

—Amy Ahlers, bestselling author of *Big Fat Lies Women Tell Themselves*

"*Adventures for Your Soul* is a breakthrough guide to help you release negative thought patterns and live a life you are in love with."

—Christine Hassler, author of *Expectation Hangover*, life coach and speaker

"Shannon is a modern thought leader on the rise!"   —CaféTruth

"Shannon Kaiser is the real deal. Her unique message hits to the core of the human spirit."   —*Healing Lifestyles & Spas* magazine

"Through her candid sharing of personal experiences and depth of understanding, Shannon is able to bring forth universal wisdom and truths in a fresh, lively voice." —*Organic Spa* magazine

"Shannon knows happiness! She not only shares the steps she took to leave depression behind, but she makes finding lasting happiness joyful. She will help you uncover your self-sabotaging habits so you break free from fear, self doubt, and lack. This guide in your hands is the key to your happy life."

—Linda Joy, publisher of *Aspire* magazine

"Shannon Kaiser, the happiness guru, writes bestselling books and wildly popular blogs about happiness, inspiring people around the world to ditch what doesn't serve them and follow their paths to true joy and satisfaction." —*MindBodyGreen*

"I've worked in the wellness industry for decades, and I've read a lot of great inspirational books. This stands out for its simple, easy-to-implement principles and honest perspective. Shannon's book is an adventure for your soul, and it will transform the way you see yourself and the world. Get ready to fall in love with your entire life!"

—Robyn Lawrence, author of *The Wabi-Sabi House: The Japanese Art of Imperfect Beauty*

Adventures *for* YOUR SOUL

21 Ways to Transform Your Habits and Reach Your Full Potential

SHANNON KAISER

BERKLEY BOOKS, NEW YORK

BERKLEY

An imprint of Penguin Random House LLC
375 Hudson Street, New York, New York 10014

This book is an original publication of Penguin Random House LLC.

Library of Congress Cataloging-in-Publication Data

Kaiser, Shannon.
Adventures for your soul : 21 ways to transform your habits and reach your full
potential / Shannon Kaiser.
p.   cm.
ISBN 978-0-425-27823-9
1. Self-realization.   2. Change (Psychology)   3. Conduct of life.   I. Title.
BF637.S4K3135 2015
158.1—dc23
2015011927

PUBLISHING HISTORY
Berkley trade paperback edition / August 2015

PRINTED IN THE UNITED STATES OF AMERICA

10 9 8 7 6 5 4 3 2 1

Interior text design by Kristin del Rosario.

Penguin
Random
House

To the best dad in the world,
Mike Kaiser.

You raised me to always follow my heart
and stay true to myself.

Thank you for your unconditional love,
unyielding support, and wise guidance.

I love you.

Contents

Foreword

by Kristine Carlson

Have you ever felt like you were just simply going to combust from the internal pressure that's been building inside you for a long time as you fill with anxiety and fear of not being able to have what you most deeply desire? Maybe you don't even know what you desire. Maybe you are so caught up in your head you can't even hear your heart. Well, no worries, there's more than hope for you here. *Adventures for Your Soul* is the book that will be your road map for change.

Scrolling through the Table of Contents of *Adventures for Your Soul*, I found myself smiling because Shannon Kaiser nailed it! You are about to embark on the adventure of your life! Shannon is one of the happiest people I know, and she will be guiding you on this journey, showing you a lighted path that will change your life.

One important thing to consider is this: We are thinking creatures, and our thinking is as automated as the breaths we take. We do it thousands of times all day long—and it's just about as invisible to us as our breathing unless we wake up and become conscious and aware of our thinking. Shannon gives you the tools you need to become aware of mental tapes that play over and over in your head and offers a solution by providing a mental makeover to help you change your habits and put you firmly on the road to happiness.

Be aware that happiness is not a pursuit, although it's tempting to think so. It appears that all of our gratification in life comes from our accolades, the way we look, and all the stuff we acquire. But no, happiness is none of these things in and of themselves. Happiness is *the journey*. And Shannon provides a "joy route" that changes the mental dynamics holding you back—not from achieving all these things but actually from receiving the JOY when you do achieve. With minds-run-wild, we are subject to being slave to habitual ways of thinking that become unconscious—meaning you might as well be sleepwalking through your life. The only way to be free of the shackles of limitation in this dreamlike state is to liberate repetitive thought patterns that undeniably self-sabotage and suffocate dreams. Muddled by too much thinking, we can easily lose a sense of the natural communication that happens between our hearts and our heads when our minds are clear. *Adventures for Your Soul* enables us to reopen that pathway and find true happiness.

I once knew a college student named Amy who was very negative and played the victim at every turn. From the outside looking in, Amy had everything. She was smart, attractive, and likable. She had a good family, and she was responsible and caring. What she lacked is the awareness that 100 percent of her anxiety and unhappiness came from inside her mind as she constantly looked for what was wrong with her life instead of focusing on the good stuff happening. Setting too high of expectations for herself and others, she lived with the resentment that follows when all things fall short of those expectations. She sometimes acted out due to the depression that followed, often pushing away the people who cared for her most. She didn't know that all of this was coming from her lack of awareness of some simple principles to happiness—the primary one being that thought precedes feelings and the emotional reactions we have to what's going on in our lives.

THERE ARE THREE THINGS YOU WILL LEARN FROM *ADVENTURES FOR YOUR SOUL*:

1. You don't have to be stuck in your fears and anxiety any longer.
2. You can recognize and reverse the habits that hinder your ability to hear the language of your heart.
3. The route you can take into your own mind to get back on the journey of joy can be a fun adventure!

Change happens from the inside out, and while many people say it, what Shannon is really pointing to is this: If you want your golden ticket onto the happiness train, you had better first understand the train of thought that you engage with may actually be taking you in the opposite direction of where you really want to go. And, well, that's like being on a train without a conductor.

What I love so much about this book is the way Shannon shows that self-awareness is the key to success in all areas of your life, whether it be your personal relationships, your career, or your optimal physical health. Shannon's inquiry of body health and its relationship to our happiness is critical to shape-shifting into the person you were born to be versus the unconscious being that is driven by invisible habits without an internal compass directing the way. *Adventures for Your Soul* will help you develop your internal compass. It points to the value of aligning mind, body, and heart to be the receiver of happiness that comes through having a joy-filled mind-set that expands our heart's deepest desire, which is to live the best life we can with maximum fulfillment.

This is precisely why *Adventures for Your Soul* is such a profound book and a must-read for anyone who prioritizes happiness as the reason why we do all things in life for others and ourselves. This is the playbook for making small changes and shifts that will yield you large results. The principles in this book will help light the path and teach you the tools for a mental makeover that will turn your scary roller-coaster ride into an adventure and joyride as you find your way back to your natural state of being—happy.

Treasure the gifts of life and love,
KRISTINE CARLSON
coauthor of the
Don't Sweat the Small Stuff wisdom book series

Adventures
for Your Soul

Introduction

Today, I consider myself an extremely happy person, but it hasn't always been that way. The truth is that I've made HUGE strides to be where I am today. I had to dig deep inside myself to access authentic joy, the kind that cannot be manufactured by false promises and one-night-stand mantras spit out by pop psychologists. I used to cry myself to sleep every night. I walked around the cold Chicago city feeling lifeless, numb, and bored with life. At night the tears would always creep aggressively back in and rock me to sleep. I would obsess over my day, and feel tremendous guilt and anxiety tied to my eating disorders, drug addictions, poor choices in men, and staying in a job I hated. These bad feelings would just push me back to my bad behaviors. I would do whatever I could to avoid the sinking feeling that I hated my life and myself, so I tried to numb myself with food, drugs, codependent relationships, etc. It was a vicious cycle.

Realizing something was wrong, I went to my doctor. She diagnosed me with clinical depression and wrote me a prescription. As I opened the door to the pharmacy, an invisible wall literally pushed me back. It was as if a force field had sprung up in front of me, preventing me from getting the prescription filled. As I looked at the scribbled piece of paper, I had an awakening. Although I knew depression is a real, serious mood disorder that requires treatment, and that for many, antidepressant drugs are necessary, my inner voice said, "This is not you; you don't need drugs to feel better. Just follow your heart." I'm not quite sure where that conviction came from. Although I believe that we all have that inner knowing of who we are and what we need, that voice had been muffled so long, drowned out with the thoughts of self-hatred that tormented me. That moment was the turning point of my life. As I ripped up the prescription, I made a promise to myself to always follow my heart and to stop making excuses for being unhappy. I realized, in that moment, that I couldn't control the world around me but I could learn how to control my own role in my life. I could continue to allow the world to happen to me, or I could happen to the world, meaning I could make a difference by becoming healthy and happy. If I could turn my pain into purpose, then perhaps this depression and these dark days could be worth it. I had a choice: I could continue to go down a path that hurt my soul, or I could clean up my life, my thoughts, and my situations. I set out on a mission to heal myself. My thought was that if one less person in the world was hurting, then that is making a difference and helping the world. So I chose to take responsibility for me. No one else, just me. And the most glorious thing happened; I became happy. I found myself. I fell in love with life.

I will be honest: It wasn't a miraculous healing or anything that happened overnight, but rather a consistent focus on showing up and taking responsibly for myself and my own life.

Over time things really fell into place. I used the tools I share in this book to help me reach a peaceful state. Finding hope and inner peace and reaching happiness is a process. But when we show up for the process, we are doing our part and that is enough. Just showing up is the largest part of the battle. And I continued to show up for myself by taking small steps to happiness. I adopted a dog (who is still my adventure buddy), who brought me immense joy through fleeting moments of pain. I moved back to the city I grew up in, Portland, Oregon, to be closer to my family; I left my job in advertising to find work that was more fulfilling, which led me to everything I do today. It was lots of small steps that led to the large transformation in my life.

Until that point of my life, fear had been controlling my every action. Fears like "I am not worthy of love," "I don't matter," "I don't make a difference," kept me playing safe. These fears were subconscious but ruling my choices in life. For example, by believing I was not worthy of love, I picked emotionally troubled men, who were controlling or drug addicts. They too supported my belief that I didn't matter. But once I saw how fear was running the show, I saw how my life had played out. I was miserable. I thought to myself, "Instead of ignoring or running from my fears, what if I dove into them?" The depression, drugs, and eating disorders were all masks keeping me from accessing my true self. Once I acknowledged my fears directly, I could see they were not real and I was able to change things. I immediately broke off my bad romance. I took the steps necessary to free me from addictions and my eating disorders. I joined support groups and twelve-step meetings and found teachers, books, and spiritual guidance to help heal these areas of my life. The right teachers and books came to me, and I was able to free myself from the troubling past. Again, it wasn't an overnight fix. I say this because a lot of the time when we get onto a self-development path, we expect instant results. And when we don't see changes, we get angry, feel guilty, or get mad at ourselves. In my own journey, I chose to take the expectations out of my healing and instead turned to trusting that each action I took would indeed help me feel happier and healthier. By being in the journey of my own life I was able to go deeper into the healing and allow the process to unfold. This meant I released all self-inflected guilt or stress, which in turn allowed me to heal faster and make smarter choices for myself.

I left my fancy corporate job in advertising to move back to the West Coast to be closer to my family. Even though I had quit my job and my romance and separated myself from the distractions of addiction and eating disorders, the journey to wellness had only just begun.

I started to trust the guidance within myself. When I first left corporate, I didn't know what I wanted to do, I just knew what I was doing was not working. I began to focus on what I wanted instead of what I didn't want. Even though I didn't know what I wanted in the grand scheme of my life, I knew that I wanted to be happy in the moment. So I focused on things, activities, and people that made me happy. I opened myself to life's opportunities and I started to sense a shift in my perspective. I began to see all things in a new light. There was richness to my life that I was previously blocked from experiencing because of my fear and depression. Small, simple things, like watching the leaves on tress blow in the wind, listening to birds sing, or turning my face to the sun to see the magnificent clouds all became incredibly joyful. I was alive. I began to celebrate the simple pleasures in life and be thankful for my own existence. I started to hear my heart again.

Each adventure I took became a spiritual awakening and a metaphor of my own existence. For example, as I pulled out my magic list (bucket list) I started to check off things like skydiving, and that became a metaphor for working through fear to reach freedom. As I started to live my life more consciously, I began to write. When I wrote about my experiences, something happened to me. I was overwhelmed with love, joy, and true peace. Writing became my sanctuary. I started to document my healing journey in articles for the local newspaper and on my blog. I wrote about overcoming fear in relation to my adventures playing with the world, like bungee jumping or skydiving. As I shared stories, readers reached out to me to say how much they enjoyed my stories. My heart felt incredibly fulfilled with each new message and story I wrote. I sent one story to *Chicken Soup for the Soul* on a whim. Not thinking much about my submission several months later, I received an acceptance letter, which read, "Congratulations. You've been selected as a feature author for our upcoming book, *Chicken Soup for the Soul: Think Positive*." I fell to the floor with excitement, and for the first time in several years, tears of happiness came flooding through. I discovered I am a writer. My greatest joy is sharing my experiences with others. Being a writer was a dream tucked in my heart since I was a little girl. I used to go outside on recess and while other kids were running around and swinging on the swing set, I was sitting in the grass with my journal, writing poetry about animals and the beautiful earth. After the fear and all the layers of pain subsided, I could return to my true self, the younger me that was always there, but just needed to be re-realized.

I began to understand that there were dreams and goals that sat quietly inside my heart, but I had been too distracted to hear them or too afraid to acknowledge and pursue them. When I was depressed, these secret dreams lay dormant and happiness evaded me. As I began to awaken to my heart's true desires and dared to pursue them, a miraculous thing happened: I felt happier and my life felt fuller. But it wasn't the achievement of these goals and dreams that led to these feelings; it was simply the journey of joy toward them. What was keeping me from pursuing my dreams, what was keeping me from moving forward in my life, what was keeping me from happiness, were my own negative thoughts. It was only when I dared to push past these thoughts and banish these beliefs that I was able to move forward on the road to fulfillment.

At our core, all of us want the same thing—to be happy and to live a truly wonderful life—though how we meet this need differs from person to person. I started to see that we could all be happier if we knew what was keeping us from happiness. Limiting beliefs and fear can stop us from moving forward in life. In many cases, we have daily habits that have become patterns which hinder our happiness. Once we know our patterns, we can break up with them if we are willing. We can understand and overcome our addiction to the suffering our self-sabotaging habits have created. These were my aha moments, and they came to me through following my joy route. The joy route is an adventure for your soul and the path to freedom, an emotional journey that we take to explore our heart's deepest desires.

Through the process of discovering my true self, I started to live my dream life. I stepped away from my life in advertising and became a travel writer, life coach, teacher, speaker, and an author. Once I tapped into the secret of the joy route, settling became impossible. My standards were raised and my dreams were being actualized.

I was on a travel writing assignment and lecturing to a group in Puerto Vallarta, Mexico, when it hit me that my next opportunity was to write about and share the process I went through to heal myself from such a dark place. Thus *Adventures for Your Soul* was born. This method is the guide I used to teach others and what I had used myself to leave a life of sadness, regret, depression, and fear behind, that had allowed me to live my dreams and travel the world sharing my message. I had already started using my life as an example to my coaching clients and workshop participants to help them heal from self-sabotaging patterns and addictions, but now I was guided to put this method into a book.

There was one small problem though . . . I was still teaching from my head. At its core, *Adventures for Your Soul* is all about the heart. And although I had already made it through extremely turbulent times, and had confidently made it through my quarter-life crisis with only a few scrapes and bruises, my real adventure had only just begun.

I was happy: I was doing work that I loved for a living and I felt fulfilled financially. My book *Find Your Happy* was doing pretty well for a first-time author. My life finally seemed to make sense and I was fully embracing my new roles of self-help author, life coach, and inspirational speaker. But although I felt joyful at times, my joy was fleeting. I recognized that I wasn't as happy as I could be.

Even though I had made great strides to improve my own life, I still felt as if something was missing. There was still a superficial layer over many of my actions. Sometimes I felt like I was just going through the motions, living but not fully alive. Upon deeper inspection, I realized there was still a lot of work to do. I was fifty pounds overweight, I was single, and I didn't feel connected to the city I lived in. I was craving a deeper connection to my own life, to my work, and to my relationships. I wasn't where I wanted to be in my life. I wanted to live somewhere where I felt part of a community. I wanted to share my life with someone special. Most of all, I wanted to feel good about myself—and I didn't. Although I knew what it meant to be happy, was I truly happy when I was self-conscious about my weight? How happy could I truly be if I stopped feeling great about myself when I looked into a mirror?

I decided to focus first on my weight since I thought that would be the easiest change to make. (Little did I realize how challenging this change would be. Nor did I realize that all my desires were linked and it didn't make sense to focus on one to the exclusion of the others.) Over a two-year period, I followed gurus, jumped on every diet trend, became a dedicated yogi, experimented with green drinks, said daily affirmations, inhaled self-help books, and went on expensive meditation retreats. Despite my efforts to achieve a more healthy body, my pants were still cutting into my stomach. Trying to reach a happy and healthy state of mind proved to be exhausting. I realized that if I continued to look outside of myself for the answers, I would probably never find them. This pivotal realization turned my searching inward.

As I looked closely at my life, I recognized idiosyncrasies and contrasts. I wanted to be healthy and love myself for who I was, but I was extremely embarrassed at all the weight I had gained. I wanted to find true love, but I was secretly afraid that no one could love me through my layers. These contradictions showed me that no amount of diets, yoga classes, and chanting with gurus would change my outcome and make me happy, healthy, and in love with my own life. I came to understand that the real change had to happen on the inside first.

Sure, we can try to make over our bodies, take part in every fad diet, wear the newest and most fashionable clothes, but without internal change, none of these makeovers will stick . . . and that is why none of my efforts were working. The real change had to be a radical new concept, and thus *Adventures for Your Soul* was truly born. I stopped focusing so much on how my life looked, and I dedicated myself to focusing on how my life felt.

The weight on my body was a manifestation of an imbalance in my thoughts. Again the fears of not being worthy, not feeling worthy of love, kept me feeling unhealthy or unapproachable. *If I wanted lasting change, I had to change the way I was looking at things and myself.* Instead of trying to change my outward environment to reach a healthy version of myself, I needed to start feeling healthy in spite of my current body shape. My change had to happen on the inside.

It wasn't my lack of willpower or lack of ability to focus on my goals that was keeping me overweight; my own limiting beliefs and emotional habits were holding me back. It became obvious that in order for me to get healthy, the emotional habits had to go. I had to look at my fears and limiting beliefs and see what they could really tell me.

The deeper I got into my internal study, the more I realized that my fears were still running the show. For example, feeling unworthy kept me in a process of overachieving (which I talk about in chapter 12, Fear Detox). I would work really hard to try to overcompensate for my insecurity of not feeling good enough.

At the same time, I discovered that I wasn't alone. I was coaching people and clients who expressed similar concerns. They wanted to be happy and healthy, but "stuff" kept blocking them from taking action. I started doing mental "push-ups," and I began practicing the steps I share in this book. As I saw positive changes in my life, I started to share my process with my clients. The results were astounding. After coaching sessions, my clients felt transformed, healed, and connected to their dreams. I too experienced transformation; I started making healthy choices and I felt more self-confident and self-aware.

Once I boldly explored my fears and used my own joy routes to remove them, I was able to accept my current conditions and more fully love myself and my life. Interestingly enough, the more I loved myself, and the more I followed my heart, the more successful and healthy I became. Once I let go of my emotional habits, my coaching practice skyrocketed, my book was selling hundreds of copies in countries all over the world, and I was invited to be featured on international radio and television shows. Best of all though, I received hundreds of personal emails from people all around the world who were empowered by my story—people who were leaving addictions, bad jobs, and relationships behind to find and live their own life adventure.

After putting myself through my own mental makeover, I realized that the size of my body and the foods that I choose to eat are part of my own creative adventure. Loving my body, no matter what size my jeans are, has been the greatest gift this work has given me.

This is not a diet book, nor is this a self-love book; it isn't even a how-to-get-happy book. (For that, check out my first book, *Find Your Happy*!) This is a book that can help you remove every obstacle in your life that is keeping you from everything you want. The tools I share in this book will help you step into what you need most for your own soul's growth. When I started this process, I thought my journey was going to be about losing weight; what I realized was that I really needed to feel good in my own skin no matter what. The gift these soul adventures gave me was a deep awakening to my own unique worth. Loving ourselves fully and living openly from our heart at every moment are the real opportunities of this journey.

Most of us have good intentions invested in making our desires a reality. We have goals we want to manifest, and we want unlimited happiness and health. The problem is that what we say and what we do about it often clash. Learning to look deeper at our intentions and our actions is what this book is about. It is a guide to help you remove the barriers that are keeping you from unlimited bliss.

Emotional habits can hurt us; they hide out and become pals with our fears, often sabotaging our best efforts to be happy. I wasn't reaching my health goals or getting what I truly wanted, because I had unknowingly brought my emotional habits along for the ride and let them limit me. I have learned that for each habit stopping us from reaching our full potential, there is a major emotional limiting belief at the root of it. For example, I recently completed thirty days in a row of hot yoga with my only goal being to lose weight. By not embracing all the other wonderful benefits

I received by sticking to the goal, I missed out on the true experience. I saw that my habit of "clinging to expectations" was actually keeping me from reaching my goals. Once I witnessed this pattern, I was able to disengage and move through my limiting beliefs. For example, I recognized I was fixating on my flaws (which I talk about in chapter 10). By focusing on what I didn't like and what wasn't working, it kept me from enjoying the journey. I learned the power of the joy route, and following my heart's true desires. Once I did this, I was able to release the insecurities and fear and be more present in the moments of my life. Which meant I showed up fully as I was in each moment.

Through my personal and coaching experiences, I have again realized that most humans are, by default, very similar. Despite differences in our cultural backgrounds, our history, or even our education, we all want to be happy. We want to have control of our lives, but we don't always know how to get it. We want to remove our fears and live successfully, abundantly, happily, and peacefully, but we keep getting stuck repeating the same patterns.

Fears about our bodies, our relationships, our jobs, the government, and the world at large affect our actions. We change our routines, switch jobs, move to different cities, buy new clothes, and try new hairstyles, diets, or relationships; no matter what we do, our fears and our patterns persist.

This book can help break that cycle. No matter what you fear, there is a process that we can use to remove the barriers keeping you from bliss. This book will delve deeply into your behaviors to help you build confidence and empower you to make healthier choices. If it helps, you can treat this book like a big "fear detox." This book will change your life if you practice the breakthrough habits shared in each section.

Today, I live and breathe the message I share in these pages and I can tell you that my life has been transformed in miraculous ways.

I am healthier, more abundant, and more fulfilled than I ever thought possible. People often tell me how I glow, and how healthy and happy I look. I am comfortable in my body, and in love with my life. Perhaps the real miracle with the principles shared in this book is that radical self-acceptance is possible. I am no longer obsessed with the numbers. I used to get on the scale, and no matter how much I gained or lost it was never enough. I would fall to the bathroom floor crying, pinching my body and screaming out in frustration, or worse, turning to food binges or purging. Today, my life is much different. The scale does not define me anymore. In fact, I use my own body for guidance. I trust myself around food, around others, and around the scale. My clothes fit better, I love what I see in the mirror, and I am genuinely happy and connected to my body. I am healthier than I have ever been.

The hard part is over; you picked up this book because something inside of you knows there is a better way. By being open and willing to make a shift, you have already given yourself permission to do the work.

This process is fun, challenging, and extremely rewarding. In each chapter I will take you through a strategic process to examine and remove the twenty-one most common emotional habits and limiting beliefs keeping you from reaching your goals. The beautiful part of the process is that this book is designed to work for you and with you; by that I mean that you can read it from start to finish as I designed it, and do the strategic exercises in each joy journey.

By understanding the key habits that are keeping you from what you truly want, you will be able to disengage from them and replace your thoughts with a new and more positive perspective. You will see a shift in your awareness, and with that awareness, your external habits will start to adjust. The weight you have been trying to lose for decades will fall away for good. Your troubled relationship with your significant other will become more loving. The job you hate and feel stuck in will change or become a thing of the past, and you will be living your passion. You will feel more connected and at peace with your best self. I know this is possible because it happened for me and hundreds of coaching clients and workshop participants.

After putting myself on this conscious cleanse and giving myself a mental makeover, my goals manifested faster. I feel healthier, and today I feel more vibrant and happy. My self-confidence has grown, and I feel completely connected to my purpose in everything I do.

If you are ready to break the habits that are holding you back for good and step into an extraordinary life, let the adventure begin!

ONE

Press the Reset Button

HABIT HINDERING HAPPINESS
We settle because we think it's the best we can get.

Many people unknowingly play it safe in order to feel love and security. Whether we take a job that does not challenge us and fails to ignite our passion, or we stay in a relationship too long, settling becomes the normal way we manage expectations and reduce pain. During my research, and from insights gleaned from multiple coaching sessions, I started to recognize a clear pattern in people's behavior. People crave new experiences and want passion in their lives, but their fear of the unknown is greater than their desire to reach that state of happiness. Fear of the unknown is one of the most common and limiting emotional habits any of us possess. It can rob us of our dreams.

Throughout this book I will share examples of each habit that hinders our happiness from my own personal experience and multiple coaching clients, and from workshops and events. As I share examples, please feel free to put yourself into the example, as most of these experiences are universal.

I thought about calling this chapter "My Move to Hawaii, and Why We Shouldn't Settle," but it wouldn't have matched the structure of the other chapters. The reality is, I recently made a huge life transition and moved to Hawaii to finish this book and in doing that I realized the power that settling can have over us if we are not aware of its power. When we settle we sacrifice ourselves, and in doing this we hurt our authentic connection with others.

I recognized my own tendency to settle in multiple areas of my life. I would settle in romantic relationships, sacrificing my own desires in an effort to keep the relationship on balanced ground. When I was in the corporate world, after I realized the work was unfulfilling, I settled by staying in the environment. Even in the places I chose to live I would settle. Maybe you can relate. Is there an area of your life where you feel restricted or bored? Many of us are unaware that we are settling because we are so used to going through the motions. Most of us are just doing the best we can to survive. But I want you to thrive, and in thriving we must look at the habits blocking us from accessing our joy. Settling is the default habit we fall into because it is safe and keeps us feeling secure.

The most prominent and recent example in my own life was settling in my environment. In both my physical environment, living in Portland, Oregon, and my own physical body, I was uncomfortable.

When I first left my corporate job, I came back to my hometown in Oregon. Spending time with family was essential for my healing and regrouping as I stepped into my new career as an author and life coach. But as time went on, I started to gain even more weight and became increasingly isolated, never really wanting to go out or do things. I realized I did not feel comfortable in the city I lived in, and my depression started to creep back in.

My "enough epiphany" came when I noticed that even though I was close to my family and childhood friends, I still felt alone and sad. That is when I learned the importance of our environment and that where we live can have a profound effect on our own happiness. If we don't like our environment or feel connected to it, we can't feel fully connected to our best self. In the process of settling for my environment, I piled on over thirty pounds. I was denying my own true self-happiness by staying in a less-than-supportive situation.

I was not inspired by my location, and this had a huge impact on my health, physically, emotionally, and spiritually. When we settle in life, it can manifest into many unhealthy outcomes, things like depression, addictions, debt, and weight gain. These unhealthy habits become a way to manage our unmet needs; we turn to self-soothing devices like food, alcohol, shopping, or self-sabotage instead of confronting the real problem. This was the pattern I was falling into, and I knew I needed to do something before I fell too far. When I finally heard my inner voice tell me I didn't need antidepressants and that I just needed to follow my heart, I made radical changes in my life, including leaving my job and my bad relationship. I also moved back home. But the truth is, while I needed to be there initially, staying there was not the path my heart wanted to take. I was settling for a dark loft in a city that didn't fill me with joy. In turn, I was settling for an unhealthy, overweight body. When we settle, our dreams often get suffocated. My unhappiness with my environment drowned out the desires in my heart, and because I was complacent in my unhappiness and doing whatever I could just to get through each day, I didn't give myself time to think about what I really wanted. That is until things got so bad I started to cry myself to sleep again, and although I had overcome my drug addictions, I was still leaning into food; I had multiple late-night binge-fests and stopped exercising. I was ashamed of all the weight I had gained and I couldn't find motivation for life. This is what settling can do to us! It steals our joy and manifests into lack of motivation and uninspired action. This was my enough epiphany.

What is your enough epiphany? This is the moment you realize that things are so bad that the situation has to change. It's the moment when the idea of moving forward in your current state feels like torture, the moment when the only way forward is to change. It's often when our mental state is conditioned and ready to accept a new behavior or change of atmosphere. Most major transitions in life—getting married, getting divorced, buying or selling a home, moving to a new location, or just "starting over"—start with an enough epiphany. The enough epiphany can be a beautiful moment of self-discovery. Your soul says, "Enough is enough, dear. It is time to make a change," and you start moving toward what you really want.

Knowing you've reached the time for change is really the first aspect of moving out of settling. At this stage your soul is desperate for transformation.

Think about your own life and the areas where you are settling. Most of the time, when you look closely, you will find you have one or two areas of your life that could use the focus of a little more love and compassion. Looking at the situations in your life where you are settling and analyzing them on a deeper level will help you pull out of this emotional habit. We often settle because we think it is the best we can get, a behavior that is rooted in fear of the unknown or in feeling unworthy. The root cause of my settling in my life was my fear of the unknown. Portland, Oregon, was safe; my family was there. I asked myself what would happen if I moved to a place I really loved? Where do I really want to be? I dreamed of working from anywhere in the world and having a location-independent business; then why wasn't I living my dream? BAM! This revelation showed me why I was so unhappy. I wasn't following my heart, therefore I was bored with life and packing on weight.

The real by-product of settling is that we ignore our inner wisdom, the heart's pull that says there is a better way for you to live your life. And on some deep level, we know this to be true, but we don't move forward, worried we will make a wrong turn or be even unhappier. But the very essence to breaking this habit is to ask yourself what you really want. What is it your heart is calling you to do? Think about this in regards to the situation(s) you may be settling in. In the joy route we will go deeper, but allow yourself to ask these questions now to get warmed up.

Once I got clear about the fear driving my actions and the fact that I was ignoring my own desire to live in a place I was inspired by, I was able to recondition my mind to focus on a more loving, kind, and compassionate approach to living. For me, this approach meant asking myself where I really wanted to be. I sat down and made a list on sticky pads. Each sticky note had one desire. I wrote:

- I want to write my book in a place that inspires me.
- I want to play in nature daily.
- I want to be a great surfer.
- I want to be happy.
- I want to be in Hawaii.

There it was scribbled out on a hot pink Post-it note. I saw my heart's calling. My heart was in Hawaii. The only thing left to do was follow my heart. Now that I knew what I wanted, the next step was to take action toward it, and refuse to settle. I am not suggesting that anyone go to the extreme of uprooting their life by committing to a move to a destination in the middle of the Pacific Ocean, but look at your life and align with what you want in your heart. Maybe Hawaii isn't your goal. But everyone has a "Hawaii," a dream tucked in their heart, and when it's ignored, we self-sabotage and settle.

Once I outed my desire, my inner self guided me to take steps to put this dream into motion. I picked a date to move, and I took my dog to the vet to go through the long process of moving him to the island. I started to downsize my stuff, stripping down and removing things I no longer wanted by donating them to Goodwill. All of these actions were supported by my inner drive to reach my happiness. I focused on what I wanted instead of what I didn't want. Settling was no longer a way I could live. I made Hawaii vision boards and started to share my dream with others. The more I focused on my heart's desires, the happier I became. I felt free.

What we all long for is love and freedom. The freedom to be who we really are and express our true self. When we settle we block off the connection of showing the world our true self. This is why we feel disconnected, unsupported, and unloved. Settling hurts more than just the present way of living; it hurts our soul and keeps us from doing what we really want to do in life.

The real mission of breaking this emotional habit and freeing yourself from settling is to honor your inner voice in the moment. Honoring your inner voice will almost always lead you to press the reset button of your life.

⟋⟋

JOY ROUTE

Press the reset button of your life.

When you look deeply into your own habits, you will see the areas that are stopping you from reaching your goals. To start, ask yourself where you are settling. It could be in the job you hate. Perhaps it's the relationship that bores you. It may even be the knowledge that you are procrastinating on the path to achieving your biggest dream.

We settle in many different areas of our life, but we don't have to live this way. Imagine what your life would look like if you had everything you dream of. What would it look like if you never settled? What if you lived out your purpose and passion? I have found in my own journey that the more I changed what wasn't working, the faster I became grounded and the more comfortable I became in knowing who I really was. That just made it easier to raise my standards. Settling became a way of my past, and the habit of settling was removed completely. Once you really tap into your inner source of abundance and authentic worth, settling for anything becomes painful and impossible to do. You raise your standards and step into an extraordinary life.

In order not to settle for less in life, we must first address the fears behind our actions. If you are in a situation that feels safe, but you are unhappy, the work is to realize your greatness and welcome in the unknown. To do this, you can start to paint a new mental picture of what you want your future to look like. Don't hold back on your vision. Imagine every aspect possible. When I first moved back to Portland, I was living in a cold, dark basement apartment, but I didn't let that stop me from focusing on what I wanted. I had a desire to be a travel writer. I visualized myself in other countries, traveling and sharing my journey with others. I pictured myself sitting on the warm sand looking out into the crystal blue Caribbean Sea. The salty air stung my nose. I imagined the warm sun touching my skin and in my hand was a journal as I jotted down notes from my experience. I smelled the fresh air and visualized every detail as if it were really happening. I did this for just five minutes a day. Five months later one of the magazines I freelanced for sent me on my first official travel writing assignment to Saint Lucia. When I arrived at the hotel I walked around the property and headed to the back of the lot. As I walked past tall palm tress and gazed forward, my mouth dropped to the ground. The same image I had been visualizing in my mind was right in front of me in real time. You see, our mind doesn't know the difference between real and fake. If you imagine something in your mind and dedicate yourself to your vision (even just five minutes a day) you will see your dream realized.

I often ask my life-coaching clients to describe their ideal life to me. At first it is often difficult, because many of us spend so much time forcing on what isn't working or what our current situation is. But to break free from the emotional pain, turn your attention to what you want by focusing on the feelings. My visualization was complete because I felt the warm air on my skin, I felt the freedom of being able to work from anywhere in the world. I felt the essence of my ideal life. You may not know exactly what you want, but you do know how you want to feel. Focus on the details of your ideal life by including your ideal feelings.

Don't worry if your present life looks nothing like your dream life. You can press the reset button on your life at any time. Give it a try. Spend a couple of minutes really homing in on your ideal scenario. Focus on the feeling and allow yourself to dream a little. By visualizing yourself as a successful, happy, and healthy person, it can come to you faster. As you focus on resetting your life, you focus on what you want instead of what you don't want. Catch yourself and your thoughts and redirect them to your ideal future. Many people say, "Yes, that's well and good, but that's not my current situation. I may want to be wealthy, but I don't know how I will pay the bills that are due right now. Or sure, it's nice to think about being in a healthy body, but my doctor told me I am in danger of high cholesterol and I have diabetes now." The future is tomorrow, but now is the problem. If you feel this way, recognize that the visualization method is a tool to help you attract what you truly want. What you experience today is only temporary.

Nothing is permanent; at every moment of your life you have an opportunity to change directions. Resetting your life is really raising your standards. The real problem in our fear of the unknown and in our feelings of unworthiness is not that we want to feel safe, although that drives us. It is the notion that we don't trust the universe to give us what we really want. When we don't feel worthy of getting great love, or we don't feel capable of excelling at our dream job, we may settle into a familiar, though not very comfortable, reality.

Fear can block your financial, physical, spiritual, and personal abundance. Looking at the patterns of our lives, we can begin to shift our limiting beliefs. To do this, you can start by feeling the vibration of what you really want. Everything has a vibrational frequency. Love is the highest energetic frequency and fear is—yes, you guessed it—the lowest. This means that you need to focus more on what you want rather than what you don't want. It means mentally creating a new reality by literally resetting your direction.

One way to do this is to visualize. Imagining yourself in a better situation, where you are happy and healthy, living in abundance, is a good way to break away from the comfortable scenery of playing it safe. Albert Einstein said, "Imagination is more important than knowledge." Imagination is where the radical reset happens first. Give yourself permission to dream about a better life. You see, many of us don't know what we want at first. I didn't know Hawaii was my dream until I sat down and started to dream out loud. Then as I went through the process, it unfolded rapidly and my heart was leading the way.

I played the "What if . . . ?" game: "What if I lived in Hawaii, and woke up by the sea every day?" "What if I actually put my dreams into motion and let myself feel expansive?" The "What if" game is the first step to getting out of your own way and living a life you are in love with, sans settling.

For this joy route we can take cues from Hollywood. Using the metaphor of a movie can help us bust through our own blocks and never ever settle again. Just like the characters of a movie, you are a character in the show called "Life." Are you in a starring role?

Or are you a supporting actor? If you are settling in life, chances are you are supporting others and putting their needs ahead of your own. When we settle for anything, our experience of living life fully is restricted. This joy route will align you with your internal compass so you will feel expansive and alive.

AWESOME ACTION 1: Write Out Your Blockbuster Hit

To prevent yourself from settling, start to see your life as a blockbuster hit. Look at the cast of characters in your life and see who is supportive and uplifting and who are the villains. Put yourself in the starring role. In your movie, others shouldn't be making decisions for you, nor should you be sacrificing your own self for the needs of others. A reader of my first book, *Find Your Happy*, reached out after reading it and said she used to be full of a lot of fear. The old her would let everyone make decisions for her. But after putting herself in the starring role of her own life movie, she realized she wanted to buy a Harley-Davidson and be a badass biker chick. After years of being an "extra" or supporting role in her own life story, she wanted to break out, and that meant stepping into the person she really is deep inside, the confident queen who craved open-road freedom. When you put yourself in the starring role of your own life, miracles happen; you become happy and full of inner peace. Some things may surprise you, but go with it because when your heart is your compass, you are full of love and light. This light is infectious for all around you. When you truly step into your true desires and live them, settling will be a thing of your past. My moving to Hawaii was an example of me starring in my leading role of life, and this breakthrough move was a pivotal moment in my character's outcome.

Look at yourself as a character of a movie and pull out your joy journal (your journal can be a special notebook or a document on your computer—the choice is yours) and answer the key questions below.

Joy Journal Freewrite:
Write Your Blockbuster Hit

1. If your life were a movie, and you were the leading character, how would you want to be portrayed?
2. If all circumstances allowed (you had enough time and money), what would you really want to do? How would your movie play out?
3. What is your happy ending? What desires are in your heart that want to be freed?
4. Where does your story take place? What location? What is the environment like?
5. What does your ideal life look like?

AWESOME ACTION 2: Press Play

Any area of your life where you are settling can be reset by recognizing *why* you are settling. What needs are being met by things being the way they are? Everything we do is motivated by a need, so your current circumstances must be fulfilling some need. Are you afraid of the unknown and your present situation feels safe? Are you afraid of failing if you attempt to reach your goals? Are things just easier because change would disturb others and you want to avoid conflict? Try to home in on what need is fulfilled by settling, and then try finding other ways to meet that same need but that are aligned with your dreams. When you do this, you are pressing the play button of your life. Just like you press play to watch a movie, you press the play button to your own dreams. After writing out your script and plan for your bestselling blockbuster life hit, play it out. Start living out goals and dreams by playing your way into new opportunities. Play is about trying things and releasing the expectations of the outcome. My journey to Hawaii was a desire inspired by my own heart, but I let go of the outcome, I released the need to know if it was the right or wrong choice for me, and instead I allowed myself to be fully in the moment. This meant I played my way to happiness. Of course once I arrived in Hawaii I loved it even more than I expected, but there was no way for me to know if this was a right choice for my big picture unless I tried it out first and pushed the play button of my life. I let go of the outcome, which allowed me to be present in the journey.

Press play on your dreams and watch your world open up into new possibilities.

For the next thirty days, give yourself permission to press the play button of your life. That dream inside your heart, the one that keeps popping up, is ready to be actualized.

Joy Journal Freewrite: Press Play

1. How can you put your dream into action?
2. What steps can you do to press play on your dream life?
3. Where do you feel like you are settling or working really hard to make something happen? Can you take a more compassionate or playful approach?

AWESOME ACTION 3: Action, Baby

Get your director hat on and get ready to say ACTION! Take action on your life. This means after you write out your life script and start to play your way to happiness, you actually take action on tangible goals. For example, my move to Hawaii didn't happen overnight; it was a clearly thought-out plan that was rolled out and executed with care and focus. Execute your **life plan** with care and focus. You do that by setting up clear steps **to help** you reach new goals. Once you start to put your real desires into focus, you will see that there are baby steps you can take to move you toward fulfillment.

For me, this meant I had to get clear about what islands I wanted to go to and how long was I going to stay in Hawaii. Was it better for me to move there in one step, or move for a few months to see which island I liked best and then move my stuff over? Once I answered my questions, I put a plan into action. This meant picking a date, arranging for places to stay on each island, etc.

When we first move away from settling, it can sometimes feel overwhelming. You may be so used to settling in your life that when you start to plan out your ideal life, it can be unnerving to realize all the actions and steps you need to take to get you where you want to go. The golden rule I tell clients and use in my own life is to not take action until you are ready.

Note: If it feels right, take a step; if it doesn't feel right, wait until it feels right. You can't rush your dreams; they have a divine order to them, and letting them unfold naturally will help you live with more joy. So how do we differentiate between really not being ready and fear holding us back? For that, ask yourself how much resistance you feel. As Steven Pressfield says in his book *The War of Art,*

> *Resistance is experienced as fear; the degree of fear equates to the strength of Resistance. Therefore the more fear we feel about a specific enterprise, the more certain we can be that that enterprise is important to us and to the growth of our soul. That's why we feel so much Resistance. If it meant nothing to us, there'd be no Resistance. Are you paralyzed with fear? That's a good sign. Fear is good. Like self-doubt, fear is an indicator.*

*Fear tells us what we have to do. Remember one rule of thumb:
the more scared we are of a work or calling, the more sure we
can be that we have to do it.*

With that said, there is always something you can do to help
you get closer to your goal. Go inward and ask yourself the following questions:

JOY JOURNAL FREEWRITE: ACTION, BABY

1. What steps can I take to action out my goal?
2. Can you call someone who will help give you more information?
3. Can you put a deposit down?
4. Can you buy a book on the subject that will help you get clearer
   on the process?
5. Can you research alternate options for reaching the goal?

AWESOME ACTION 4: Sit Back and Enjoy the Show

The fun part has arrived: Sit back and enjoy the show. That's right.
Your life is like a movie and it is played out on the big screen. At
some point all of your hard work and effort come together to create a state of flow. The state of flow is like the movie premiere. You
get to sit back and relax as your dreams manifest and become a
way of your normal life. Just like enjoying a movie on the big screen,
you have to enjoy your own life. The efforts you put forward in
your life can be achieved, but if they are not enjoyed along the way,
it makes it hard for you to manifest more abundance and joy. Since
my arrival in Hawaii, I have been on an abundance adventure of
sitting back and enjoying my own show. At the start of this movie,
I was depressed, overweight, and settling. Once I put all of these

joyful steps into play, I became my own hero by discovering my heart's true desire. I made my dreams come true by focusing on a plan and then actualizing it. Since arriving in Hawaii, I have been on what feels like one long vacation, but this is my life. This is the equation of all of my hard work, passion, and trust coming together to create a life I love. This is me feeling grateful for working and playing in one of the most beautiful places on earth. I let my life play out in a way that inspired me. And this can happen for you. Do not settle in life; it will make you feel horrible inside. What you want is to feel joyful, expansive, and in love with life. And this only happens when you take a stand for yourself and become your own main character of your own life. Let your movie unfold naturally and have fun directing your own life show.

When you press the reset button of your life, you can change the fate of your future, and settling will become a way of your past.

MOTIVATIONAL MANTRA

To truly break this habit, carry this mantra with you. In any moment when you find yourself settling, repeat these powerful words.

"I can change the fate of my future.
Settling is the way of my past.
I do not settle."

TWO

Break Up with Your Issues

❧

HABIT HINDERING HAPPINESS

We stay victims to the harassment of our life.

Here is the first blog post I ever posted publicly:

After grinding second gear, I glare down. "Crap!" Fresh green juice is splashed all over my silk blouse. I am already late for work and extremely irritated because I won't have time for my morning savior, Mr. Starbucks. As if that wasn't the end of my day, I am stuck behind the slowest school bus in the universe. Every twenty feet bright red lights flash out and warn me to STOP, almost challenging me to unlawfully pass in order to follow through with my day. I am yelling in my head about how bad things are going, and mentally abusing myself because I didn't even have time to brush my hair. My makeup looks like I was drunk when I put it on, and I didn't work out this morning as I intended to do last night, so I am feeling bloated and uncomfortable from last night's extra helpings of food. I take a deep breath in, and release. Then I become even more annoyed because that didn't even help.

Once again the giant stop sign flings out, and as the giddy children bounce on the bus to embrace their glorious day I see a pattern in all of them. They are all consumed with unbounded excitement, as if the world is their playground and it starts when they get on that school bus. In this moment I realize that I am causing my own distress. The racket in my mind is a feeding ground for my ego, and I am eating up every bite of its adrenaline-pumped poison. As I watch the stop sign pop out yet again, I conclude that it is the universe's way of telling me to literally "STOP!" slow down and appreciate my day. I close my eyes briefly, and say, "Anger, I see you, I feel you, and I release you." Then I ask for a miracle and release it to the universe. Within moments, we come to a stoplight. I glance up from my self-induced pity party and see a young boy in the backseat of the bus enthusiastically trying to get my attention. As we lock eyes, he raises his hand and flashes me a peace sign coupled with a giant goofy grin.

I smile back as my silly stresses disappear. As you might guess, that was my miracle. The angels appointed that little boy the messenger, delivering a message I so desperately needed to receive. It was as if that little boy was saying, "Lighten up, lady, and just smile more." I got the message loud and clear: We must always practice peace in our hearts toward ourselves and to others. And more importantly we can't always control what happens in our life, but we can control how we react.

Maybe you can relate to my story. I wrote this blog many years ago, a week before I left my corporate job and was struggling to find my purpose and passion for life. Every day was a constant game of catch-up and trying to get ahead, but one thing after another would push me back and keep me miserable, angry, and depressed. That is, until I slowed down and released my silly stress. After I put things into perspective, it became clear to me that I was staying victim to the harassments in my life, letting life situations dictate my mood, my outlook, and my life.

Many of us have situations in our life that happen, perhaps unexpectedly, and we focus our attention on the situation and how bad things turned out, which creates a snowball effect of more drama and chaos. Like attracts like, which also means that negative energy attracts negative energy. Think about the hiccups in your life. We have all had days where we are stuck in traffic, spill our coffee, are late for a meeting, lose our keys, stub our toe, can't fit into our jeans, miss important deadlines, get rejected, have car issues, health problems, and life just keeps throwing dirt in our face. Despite it all, we plunge forward, trying to escape the madness . . . and then even more crazy hits the fan. This is called Crazy Town, and most of us have moments, days, even weeks, months, and years when we feel like permanent residents of Crazy Town. Those times when one bad thought from a situation latches on to another and all of a sudden we are paralyzed by the harassment of our lives. We fall victim to the situations in our life and it is impossible to move forward. We feel like we are just trying to dodge life's punches and stay above water.

A great example of this is my father. My dad is a tree farmer, and he lives in a beautiful home with my mom on twenty acres of farmland. Living in the country has its perks, but farm life is not for the faint of heart. Growing up on the farm, I remember my dad constantly being frustrated with crazy situations, aka Crazy Town. Situations like the sprinklers were broken, the power would go out, the tractor broke down, the deer rubbed all the bark off the trees and he lost precious inventory, woodpeckers pecking on the house . . . the list would go on and on and grow larger each day. Every single day, a new problem would arise and my father would have to roll up his sleeves and fight once again against the harassment of his life. As a teenager growing up in this environment, not only did this show me that farm life is tough, but it showed me a lot about my father and how many of us can get caught up in everyday life troubles.

I love my dad dearly, and this book is dedicated to him, but I noticed something that seemed to perpetuate the farm life disasters. With each situation my dad would encounter, he would always come into the house and say, "If it's not this, it's something else, it's always something; I can't get a break!" This is a belief and thought pattern he kept carrying around with him. Based on the results of his life, the issues associated with owning a farm and home in the country, he had conditioned himself to expect problems. He kept telling himself he couldn't get a break, so life kept giving him "broken" things to fix. This created drama and built up resentment. This resentment carried through to his work and he felt like he was always playing catch-up. My father was a victim of the harassment of his life.

Can you relate? Are there thoughts that keep popping up into your head about situations in your life? It is important to become aware of our thoughts about the situations in our life and to recognize when our beliefs are playing into the outcome. We will always attract what we believe. If you believe the world is a harsh, mean place, you will find yourself the victim of harassment or bullying. You may see more bad in the world than good, and your reality will support your beliefs. On the flip side, if you believe the world is a kind, loving place, you will see evidence of this in your everyday encounters. Strangers will smile at you, you will find parking spots up close to the store entrance, and you will feel abundant and happy. What we believe on the inside is always manifested on the outside. Pay attention to your thoughts and how they create your reality.

If you want to change your results, you need to change the way you are thinking about your results. Instead of looking at the situations in your life as problems, begin to shift your perspective to see that they are just pathways. All situations serve as a path to greater understanding to help you grow and learn more about yourself.

To avoid being victimized by the harassment of your life, you must be accountable and recognize that you are not a victim. This can be a tough pill to swallow, but consider that the experiences you are going through are part of your own creation. Yes, your own creation! No, I'm not telling you to blame yourself for all the seemingly bad things that happen in your life. That's all you need—one more thing to feel bad about! But stay with me for a moment and consider this: What if you design everything in your life, the good, the bad and the terrible? If this were true, you would be able to re-create your world for good in the same way you have created your current situation. If there are areas in your life that are not working, believe that you can change them by focusing on what you want to happen instead of what you don't want.

There is something else you can do: Instead of seeing all of the situations as bad, what if they are just neutral happenings? The things we experience in life happen, but it is up to us how we perceive them. We designate things as "good" or "bad"; we label situations and then respond accordingly. What if we could stop this labeling and take things as they come, not assigning value, letting go of negative perceptions?

Let's look at my dad's behavior as an example. He would always expect bad things to happen, and when they happened he would focus on how bad things were happening. Our negative beliefs can become a self-fulfilling prophecy. My father believed farm life was tough, therefore situations would occur daily to reinforce his belief.

He took each situation and allowed it to get the best of him. It felt like him against the world, and that those bad situations, breakdowns, and problems were always just around the corner. As you can imagine, walking around expecting bad things to happen, focusing on the negative, didn't make for a joyful life.

But then something shifted for him, and I saw a change in him. He broke up with his issues, and you can too. You too can break the habit of feeling victimized by the harassments of your life.

~

JOY ROUTE
Break up with your issues.

The shift happened in my dad when he started to look at his life on the farm in new ways. Instead of looking at the problem, he and my mother shifted to appreciation and to a focus on what was wonderful about farm life. They are living in their dream home, have multiple acres for the dogs to run leash free, and they are surrounded by abundant wildlife, birds, and fresh, clean air. They have trees they grow with love and sell to people to help make their homes more balanced and peaceful.

When my parents started to wake up each day with gratitude, they detached from the daily drama. Instead of focusing on the issues, they held space for laughter, life, and love. Problems still happened, but there were less of them, and those that did occur were not as troublesome. You see, issues are part of life, but the drama around those issues is optional. Break up with your issues. The joyful way to stop feeling victimized in your life is to actualize your gratitude. Replace your worries about what could go wrong with what could go right, and watch how your life unfolds. It will unfold beautifully and you will feel abundant, happy, and free.

Last winter I agreed to house-sit for my mother and father when they went on vacation. Just before they left, "stuff happened": one of the farmhands rammed the farm truck into a ditch by mistake, the water pipe in the house broke, and the pipes outside were about to freeze from a snowstorm. The old drama king, the one who was a victim to the harassment of his life, would have been upset, and mad at the world. He would have felt like he couldn't get a break, no matter how hard he tried, and that he just couldn't get ahead. To my surprise, when he walked in the house, he gave my mother a big hug, kissed her, and said, "Let's go on vacation!" The issues of the farm didn't affect him at all. He carried on with his life and welcomed in the awesome adventure ahead—a romantic getaway with my mom. You see, when we break up with our issues, we can create more space to welcome in what we really want in life. When we let go of what is not working, we make room for what is working. The happy, carefree, detached dad was not complaining or avoiding responsibility, he just adopted a new perspective—one of love and happiness—instead of fear and worry.

He wasn't in denial. He wasn't pretending that things didn't happen. He just realized the truck and the pipes would get fixed. He could complain and moan and mope about it first and then get them fixed, or he could skip the dramatics and just arrange for them to be fixed and get on with the flow of life. He chose the latter and was better off for it. My mom was happier, and I felt more peace watching how happy they were as they left for a romantic weekend.

You can choose to break up with your issues. This is about being in the flow of life and letting things happen as they will. If you have ever been in the ocean and tried to swim in the waves, you may have been knocked over and pushed around as you fought against them. However, if you swim like professional surfers, you dive into the wave and come out feeling refreshed, unscathed, and in the flow. Surfers ride the waves, moving along with the natural flow of the water. Life is like swimming in the ocean: We can either fight against the waves, looking at our problems as giant harsh waves, crushing us and pulling us under, or we can dive into our life and accept the natural flow. Trust me, it is much easier to go with the flow. But notice that diving in can be the scary part. When we spend our life focusing on what isn't working, and amplifying our problems, making the switch to dive in will be a little scary at first, but if we take the leap, we will find that life's harassments will no longer be weighing us down.

As I've said, the only way to stop allowing ourselves to be victims of life's harassment is to break up with our issues. Like a breakup with a romantic partner, initially this could be messy, frustrating, scary, and heartbreaking. But deep down we know that in the long run, both breakups and breaking up with our issues will save us from more pain, misery, and from settling. Breakups force us to reconsider the direction we are going in life and help us take stock of what is truly important. Although there is no really wrong way to go through a breakup, only time can heal the open wounds. When we give ourselves time, the initial shock will subside and we will relax into our new lifestyle. The same is true for breaking up with your issues. Sometimes the best way to go about a breakup is to rip off the Band-Aid or quit cold turkey, which is the approach we will take here. But don't worry; the breakup plan we will create will be based in a joyful, compassionate approach. This will help you recognize that your issues don't define you, and remind you that you are not your problems.

A couple of years ago, I visited the guru John of God in Brazil. While I was there, I received a miraculous healing, although I didn't know it at the time. I was in an organized group with thirty other travelers. Every single one of them underwent invisible surgery—a spiritual surgery the guru performs to give the human body rest, so it can recover and heal. Everyone except me. I was very concerned that I wasn't being asked to rest like my fellow travelers. I traveled over four thousand miles to the remote town of Abadiânia to see this miraculous man and I wanted to be healed like those around me. I wanted to be fixed. Why wasn't he fixing me like he fixed everyone else?

One afternoon while the rest of the people in my group were locked in their rooms fast asleep in recovery, I was antsy, so I ventured to the healing center. I meditated and got the message, loudly and clearly, that there was nothing wrong with me. I was trying so hard to be fixed, and I wanted my insecurities to miraculously float away. I desperately wanted to be healed, but there was nothing to heal. I was complete as I was. The pain and struggles in my life were not problems but pathways to greater understanding of my own heart. I was looking at my situations, the harassments of my life, as big problems. I identified with them as if they were me and that I was broken. I felt pain and that I needed to be fixed. My healing was the realization that there was nothing wrong with me. And I share this story because I want to tell you that there is nothing wrong with you. There is nothing to fix. You are not broken.

This story was a turning point in my journey to self-love. I realized that we have a choice; we can look at events in our life and see them as problems that hinder us and keep us from what we want, or we can choose to see them as opportunities for growth. We can surround our problems with love. Which one feels more loving and peaceful? The second path is often the road less traveled, but it is a beautiful road that is paved with love, inner peace, and unlimited joy. We come to realize that life doesn't happen *to* us; life happens *for* us. Every event in life is an opportunity for growth. It is our decision to see it as such.

The very first step in this joyful route is to recognize that you are not your problems.

AWESOME ACTION 1: Break Up with Your Issues

Similar to when you go through a breakup with a person, you may fall into blaming the other person or blaming yourself. If you have been dumped, or even if you are the dump-ee, it is easy to fall into blame. When it comes to breaking up with your own issues, you have to detach from blame as well. If you blame your life outcomes on the problems you face, it is essential to remove your attachment to the problems. You are not your problems. They do not define you, and you are not cursed. These situations in your life are part of a bigger picture that will unfold into your ultimate life plan. By shifting your focus away from the problems and turning to the solutions, you will have more drama-free days.

Marie Forleo, entrepreneur, my business coach, and marketing maven, always says we have reasons or we have results. Do you have more reasons or are you seeing tangible results?

To break up with your issues, think about where you are spending most of your energy. Is it on the reasons why things aren't working for you and why you can't get ahead in life, or is it on the results—how things are moving forward and dreams that are actually coming true?

When we hang out with reasons, we are stuck in victim mode. We focus on why things aren't happening, how life is unfair, and how we just can't get a break. To break up with this habit, focus your attention on the results. Pull out your joy journal and answer some fun questions.

It might be tempting to skip over these questions, but I promise, as with all of the exercises in this book, the more you put into it the more you get out of it. Do yourself a favor and take time to answer these important questions; they will guide you to freedom. These questions will help you go deeper.

1. What are the top three reasons you use that are holding you back?
2. What three steps will you take to focus on the results instead of the reasons?
3. What tangible results do you see in your life?

REPEAT THE MOTIVATIONAL MANTRA

"I am not a victim of my reality.
I consciously create joy-filled experiences."

AWESOME ACTION 2: Appreciate the Pain

The next phase of breaking up with this habit hindering our happiness is to go into each situation or problem in our lives and appreciate it. Yes, you read that correctly. Appreciate the pain. Much like a real breakup, instead of hating or regretting the relationship, the fastest healing comes from appreciation and respect for the time shared. If you are struggling with situations in your life, focusing on why it is happening can keep you playing small; when you focus on "Why me?" you are not able to move forward in life. But turning your attention to the situation and appreciating it can create miracles in your life. Try it out here: Take a situation in your life right now that is causing you a lot of emotional stress.

1. Go into the situation and say, "What can I learn here?"
2. Send love and light to the situation.
3. Repeat the words "I am thankful for the opportunity to grow and learn through this situation; I see the situation as a pathway not a problem."

AWESOME ACTION 3: Focus on the Big Picture

When we go with the flow, we suddenly recognize that everything is in the right order. Your life begins to open up as you relax into the rhythm. Each problem that comes your way will no longer feel like such a large speed bump. You will begin to focus more on your quality of life and be present in the moment. This can happen when we focus on the big picture. Think of yourself as a Hollywood movie director; just as a director has to focus on the grand scheme of things, the big picture is the overall storyline of the movie, not just one scene. The big-picture plan for your life is all about taking a step back and seeing the bigger picture at play. You are right where you need to be in order to get to where you want to go. To focus on what's not working can hinder your happiness. Instead, focus your attention on your future and the plans you want to be actualized.

The big picture is the big plan for your life that will help you move forward with more ease.

Try it out, for the next seven days.

When a situation arises, work on taking it in stride and say to yourself, "This is not happening to me, it is happening for me." With each situation, ask yourself, "What is the big picture here?" Be open to receiving guidance to help you move through the situation. For example, if you get a flat tire on your way to a job interview and are late for your meeting, instead of looking at the situation as bad, say, "Things don't happen to me, they happen for me. It is what it is. What is the big picture here?" Perhaps later you will find out that they gave the job to another person and maybe you learn that the company is going under. Your soul was helping you. Or you didn't really want that job anyway; it was not in alignment with what you really want in a job and you were going for it out of feelings of desperation and hopelessness.

No matter what the immediate situation looks like, remember there are always things happening behind the scenes. Much like a Broadway play or Hollywood movie, things are going on behind the curtain: actors prepare to go on stage, makeup is being applied, lights are adjusted, the director gives direction. Behind the curtain things are always happening, the same way the universe is working behind the scenes to get you what you want. We must trust that the show will go on. Because it always does.

The above example about getting a flat tire on the way to the job interview? That actually happened to me many years ago. Instead of looking at the flat tire with a "Why me?" attitude, I said, "This is happening for a reason." I later found out that the person I was interviewing with worked his employees super hard, the company was having financial issues, and the employees weren't getting paid. Yikes, I almost walked into that! You see, when you look at the big picture, you can see that the universe is always protecting you, that the universe is ultimately helping you. Look at situations in your life as pathways instead of problems, and you will move through life easily and with confidence.

MOTIVATIONAL MANTRA

"Things don't happen to me,
they happen for me."

THREE

Free Your Feelings

◦⌒ℯ

HABIT HINDERING HAPPINESS
We trust advice from our head, not our heart.

One of the most common habits we fall into that can hinder our happiness is overthinking things and failing to act. This shows up in the form of overanalyzing, being extremely critical, or not trusting our own feelings. In other words, we trust advice from our head more than our heart. One of my regular coaching clients described this scenario perfectly when she said that she and her best friend joke that she has a squirrel in her brain that works overtime. He runs around on a wheel overthinking everything, always overdoing, and running in circles not going anywhere. The little guy is exhausted, on crutches, and stressed out because he has worked so hard and long on "trying to figure things out."

Although we laughed about this metaphor, the reality is that most of us have a "little squirrel" in our brain that works itself into exhaustion. We worry about outcomes, we overthink situations, and we listen to every bit of advice we have consumed, which often pulls us in multiple directions. We lean into the knowledge of our brain and past experiences versus trusting our initial gut instinct. This chapter is about giving the little squirrel a break, so you can feel more joy and confidence in all of your decisions.

Imagine never having to overthink anything ever again! What would you do with all your time if you trusted that things would work out? Life can be pretty sweet when you access the inner guidance system built inside your heart.

Meet my brother. He is in information security, which is a job that works behind the scenes to protect important data stored online and in technology databases. His mission is to ward off online phishers and scammers and prevent corruption to important files and information. He prevents the "bad guys" from accessing data and planting viruses online. Essentially, he is a tech guru that protects your personal information stored online from getting into the wrong hands. This is a job that requires him to think through multiple scenarios to ensure he overcomes any and all obstacles. In order to fight off Internet crime, he has to visualize problems and threats before they arise. He thinks and solves problems before they even happen. He must be smarter than the problems that arise and the people who are trying to infiltrate his networks. This job is perfect for him and anyone who loves to analyze and think through situations.

Yet even with his decades of training and his vast store of knowledge, there are still times that a new problem arises and the knowledge stored in his head, combined with years of personal experience and education, fails him. No matter what he tries, he can't think his way out of the problem. At those times, he must feel his way out. This is when my brother's gut instinct will kick in. Using his intuition and inner guidance, he is able to solve problems that he has never encountered or considered before. Of course knowledge is essential to have in order to help solve problems, but sometimes knowledge isn't enough. New problems need new solutions; when you try to solve new problems with old solutions, you won't see results. Relying solely on knowledge and ignoring our intuition is a fast track to Rut-ville. At some point, listening to our head instead of our heart will keep us from moving forward in life.

The same is true for each of us and the problems we encounter in life. We can try to use everything we know to solve a problem, but sometimes we need to trust everything we feel. If we only listen to our head, and ignore our heart, we'll get stuck and be unable to move forward in life. Solving problems in life can become easier when we access the advice stored in our heart. There is a place where knowledge and gut feeling collide. But many of us have spent so many years trusting our heads that we are out of touch with our own instincts. Sure, you have heard people say listen to your intuition, and that your gut knows the way, but how often do we really listen to it? What does it really mean to listen to your gut instincts anyway? Why is it so hard for so many of us to access that inner voice?

I think life coach and bestselling author Martha Beck nailed it when she said that the problem is that no one has taught us what an instinctive hunch looks like. Plus, we spend our entire lives trying to override intuition; we're told to "think things through" and "to really think about our decisions." But instinct has nothing to do with thought . . . it's all about feelings, and many of us don't spend much time with our own feelings, so we haven't learned to trust them.

But trusting our heart is essential to our well-being. When we rely on thoughts alone, we can get trapped in a web of negativity. Many of our thoughts are fear based, and we wind up acting from a place of fear rather than moving forward on our best path. Or our thoughts are rooted in our low self-confidence, and we paralyze ourselves with self-judgment and self-criticism. In my private and group coaching sessions, one of the first questions I ask people is, "What are your thoughts around the situation that is causing you the most stress?" In almost every situation, my clients will pause, ponder, and say in a dismal voice, "Well, they are not good." And this is the real problem. You see, we associate the thoughts we think with our identity. We think that because, for example, we have the thought that we are fat, then we ARE fat, and that makes us feel unworthy and unlovable. Our thoughts play into our actions and choices. The tricky little bugger here is that **whatever you believe about yourself on the inside is manifested on the outside.** So if you are telling yourself you are fat all the time, then your body can become a reflection of these thoughts.

This is exactly what happened to me. On my journey to happiness and finding inner peace, I felt happy in every area of my life except with my own body. I would be so mean to my own body; I would tell it I hated it. I would cry at night, squeezing my fat rolls, pinching them so hard I would get red marks and bruises. I hated my body with such disgust; I loathed it. Plus, everything that wasn't going well in my life I blamed on my body. I didn't make the dance team in high school because of my weight. That man never called me back because of my body shape. My body was easy to blame because I didn't like it. For nearly three decades it was the scapegoat to my insecurities and unmet expectations. So many of us do this. We pick ourselves apart and blame the parts of us we don't like for things not going as well as we want. This happens because we are in our ego-based mind. Our head is making choices and dictating our direction, which means the loving heart is not consoled.

As much as I hated my body, it was still part of me, it was my flesh, so as much as I thought I was happy and teaching others how to be happy, there was a larger portion of myself that I was unhappy with and unwilling to accept. Naturally, along with this hate and resistance to accepting what was, I grew in size. The more my body grew, the less motivation I had to work out and do things to care for myself, and the cycle continued to amplify. My head was controlling the show. I trusted the advice in my head, the advice that said, "Hey, whale! Yes you, fatty, why can't you get your crap together? You are disgusting, a miserable excuse for a human." Ouch! It hurts me just thinking about how I used to talk to myself. The thoughts I felt are not that much different than the self-sabotage most of us tell ourselves daily.

My friend Christine Hassler, who is also a life coach and the author of *Expectation Hangover*, says, "If you talked to your friends the way you talked to yourself, would you have any?" Most of us treat ourselves horribly, with an overflow of negative talk inside of our head. We can analyze the self-talk and ridicule, and objectively look at what we're doing to ourselves, but we have to realize that all these negative thoughts are also felt in our heart. And in order to remove the disrespect and attacks on ourselves we need to drop into our heart and feel our love and truth. This is how I healed my relationship with myself. With respect to my body, I started to analyze the voice in my head that said, "You are so fat!" Whenever the mean words came into my head, I would drop to my heart and feel the truth. It looked something like this:

HEAD: You are so fat; you are such a giant pig.

HEART: You *FEEL* a little bloated in this moment, but you are divine and perfect as you are.

HEAD: Your pants are digging into your stomach, and you weigh more then you ever have in your life; you are hopeless.

HEART: You are full of love. You are vibrant. You are healthy.

HEAD: Hey, roller pig, put down the pint of ice cream.

HEART: What you are craving is love. Love yourself enough to fully taste this food and be present as you enjoy this loving experience.

Huge difference between the head talk and the heart talk, right? And there's no question which voice we should be listening to! Trusting yourself starts with trusting your heart and listening to it.

For most of us, the head talk is a fear voice that derives from negative projections. You may have also noticed that most of the head talk is based on assumptions from society. Cultural norms and other people's opinions will shape our internal head talk. We adopt society's standards and expectations, believing what the world says is right, and beating ourselves up when we do not live up to them. This means that if you are a woman above size 6 or 8, you consider yourself fat; or if you are above a certain age and single, you think you're a loser; or if you don't want kids, there is something wrong with you; or that if you want to take time off from work or school to travel, you are avoiding responsibility.

Well, I'm here to tell you, none of this is true, and if you dropped into your heart, you would be able to shut out the negative voice in your head and hear the words of self-love that radiate from your heart.

Embrace your body, no matter what your size! If you're single by choice, celebrate your independence; if you want a life partner but just haven't found him or her yet, don't despair, and show yourself the love you want someone else to show you. And if you have desires that "go against the grain" of societal norms, don't feel guilty; instead, realize that you have your own unique compass, and aligning with your inner desires is the only way to true joy. You can be truly happy if you align with your own heart. The depression, addictions, sadness, and hopeless emotions in our lives surface because we go against our own heart's desires. We go to war against ourselves. But when you embrace your authentic self and your desires, you will eventually fulfill your dreams. Your head will tell you that your dreams are impossible, but your heart will guide you with clarity and direction.

The advice of your head is a distorted worldview that gets funneled into your brain. This is where so much of the self-sabotage comes from. But the heart is the truth . . . your truth. Your heart knows you better than your head, because your heart is based in love. The love inside of you is real. As a *Course in Miracles* says, "Only Love is real." The inner light inside of you is your essence— the divine light that knows you are not fat or ugly or unmarriageable. Your heart knows the truth. That is why I trained myself to start accessing that truth over my fear-ridden mind-set.

We can't fully access our heart without accepting the situation that is causing us the most pain. Whether you are trying to curb overeating or find a soul mate, the key is accepting where you are right now in your journey. We must accept where we are before we can move to where we want to be. Acceptance cannot happen in our brains, it must be felt in our hearts. We can try to tell ourselves to accept our situation, love our bodies, and be kind to ourselves, but it can't happen until it is truly felt. Acceptance only happens with a full surrender.

I had to learn to surrender to what is, and disengage from the negative thoughts that said I was ugly and fat. I had to train myself to drop to my heart even in the moments of self-hate. It was in those moments, moment by moment, that the miracle could happen. The light would enter in, and I was willing to see myself in a more loving perspective. The shift happened with a surrender and willingness to let go of my attachments to my thoughts.

Once I started to release my hold on the nasty thoughts, I could feel myself more fully. The self-hate that was sitting in my thoughts was really a mask for my true feelings of vulnerability and being exposed. My body was big, so I felt open to criticism; the shame and guilt amplified. Criticism derives its power from our embarrassment and shame. If we didn't feel embarrassment and shame, other people's criticism of us or our own inner critic would have no power over us. Many of us stay stuck in self-shame, guilt, and embarrassment because we are worried about what other people will think. But when we are living from our heart, we begin to shift to love and realize that the most important thing is how we feel about ourselves.

One way we can drop from our head into our heart is to identify the difference between feelings and emotions. For example, if someone looked at me funny, I'd assume they were judging me because of my body size, and then I'd feel fat. This would make me feel sad and hopeless and depressed, but my feeling this way was actually an emotion. An emotion is a reaction to a situation or experience. Our feelings are how we feel; they are a perception of an emotion.

This emotion was still connected to my mind. I felt ashamed, but that was because I was still thinking about how the world would perceive me; it was a reaction. Feelings are not emotions. The difference between feelings and emotions is that feelings are physical. You will feel something if someone hurts you.

Emotions are the way that you assess or react to a situation. Emotions are rooted in assessing situations, whereas feelings are grounded in truth in the moment. Emotions are often in your head, whereas feelings are inspired by your body and heart. "You hurt my feelings," is an emotion, because it is based on a reaction to a situation. If someone pushed you and your body is in pain, "I am hurting" is a feeling. It is a factual result based in the moment. But if someone pushes you and you think, "They don't like me, I must be unlovable," this is an emotional assessment and reaction to the situation. Emotions create stories in our mind that are not usually true. When I felt fat and ugly, it was because I was creating the story in my mind that other people's looks at me were judgmental. I would tie this experience to the bullies from my childhood who picked on me for being a large little girl. That's the thing about emotions, they are usually tied to signatures of past events. But our feelings can change moment by moment.

What I am getting at here is that it's not what others say to us that matters, it is what we say to ourselves. And when we are living in our head, we may be more emotional or reactive, which means we assume things that aren't always true. But dropping into your heart requires a loving look at your feelings and getting in touch with them.

As I mentioned before, emotions carry energetic signatures, which means our past plays out in the present, because they are based in our thoughts or brain, whereas feelings are recognized through the physical body and tell us what is going on for us in the present moment.

Distinguishing between the two is an important step in moving forward in life with clarity and confidence. Many of us mix up our feelings and our emotions. We may say, "I feel fat," but this is an emotional response with an energetic signature. The feeling would be "I feel uncomfortable and constricted in this moment." Our head will assess: I feel fat, therefore I am fat. But our heart will prove: I feel uncomfortable and constricted in this moment, which says nothing about who I am, therefore the shame and guilt is removed. It is just what I am feeling in this moment.

Understanding the difference between the two can save you years of struggle. The foundation for a happy life is to trust your feelings and access the advice in your heart more than the thoughts emanating from your reactionary head.

By getting in touch with my feelings instead of my emotions, I could heal my self-sabotage. My head would tell me I was ugly and fat, but my heart would say, "You are just feeling this way in this moment." Learning to trust the guidance of my heart, I was able to be more compassionate with myself, which released the resistance, lightened the inner bully load, and helped me return to my natural state—one that is healthy, happy, and joyful. This process is how I started to fall in love with myself.

We trust what we think is real, and we allow these thoughts to drive our actions, but it's important to understand that what we think is not always what's real. In other words, don't believe everything you think. What we feel is ALWAYS real. Take, for example, a client I worked with who was struggling with food addiction and binge eating. She hated how much food she was eating, and no matter what she did, she couldn't stop eating. She was embarrassed at how much weight she had gained and felt jealous of people who were healthy and happy. She told me how she would see people signing up for running events and would feel a pit in her stomach, one tied to her feelings of both envy and remorse. She didn't have it in her to try to run a marathon, and this made her feel even worse about herself. She said, "I see how passionate my friends are about running, and I can't, for the life of me, understand it." She would return to her bag of potato chips and zone out in front of the TV. I asked her what her thoughts were about her binge eating. She paused, and said, "It's grim! I think, gosh, here we go again! I can't eat like a normal person. Do I even want to stop eating? Is this how my life is going to be, fat, single and alone on a Friday night?" Then I asked her, "Do you love food?" She said in an exhausted voice, "I do." So I said, "Well, great news, your problem is not a problem at all, it is a pathway. You love your food, and you are trying to tell yourself not to love it; that is the only problem." Society tells us we should not like our food, that it should be considered "bad." We resist our love of food, and then many of us will overeat and try to stuff down our desires. Why in the world would we ever hide away or deny something we love? When we do this, the resistance creates a backlash and encourages us to overeat, overdrink, overspend, and overthink everything instead of feeling. We do this because our head tells us it is bad; we are bad for eating "bad" things. But our heart knows that a little salt, a little fat, a little this, is called balance, and enjoying the foods that we love is leading a balanced life.

I encouraged my coaching client to get in touch with her feelings around her food, and to focus for seven days on fully loving her food. After a week she was blown away at the way her life had changed. She was present with her food, she thanked it, tasted it fully and appreciated every bite; her cravings died down, she stopped having episodes of bingeing and in time, just like it had with me, her weight balanced out. She was able to love her problem away; so did I, and so can you. She dropped from her head, the emotional, over-reactive part of herself, and aligned with her loving heart.

I encourage you to start listening to your heart instead of your head. By becoming aware of our thoughts, we can retrain the ego to release its hold on us. We no longer attach our self-worth to our thoughts, but we begin to trust our own heart's guidance. This can happen when we free our feelings.

JOY ROUTE
Free your feelings.

Feelings are a life-force energy that flows through you as they register a response within your physical body. Unlike emotions—which are often imposed on us by a culture that tells us what we consider good or bad, or past experiences that are coloring the present—feelings are always yours; they are yours alone. Most of the time they are brutally honest, and they urge you to take a look at what is transpiring for you in the moment. Feelings are not based on past experiences or regrets. They are not concerned about the future either. Feelings are in the moment. Accessing them and letting them have a voice is the pathway to freedom. Freeing your feelings is a learned method to help you reach more happiness.

In this joy route we will go on an inner journey to help you access your authentic feelings, not the emotions carried forward from past experiences or other people's beliefs. Remember your feelings are yours, and they are honest and raw. Allow them to be free, because they will free you of the burden of troubling situations. When we free our feelings, we allow the truth to shine.

Freeing your feelings is like entering into a dark room and turning on the light to see cockroaches scatter away. The cockroaches are the thoughts and emotions that stem from your experiences in life. They exist in the dark moments of life; when we switch on the light and turn on the truth, they have no choice but to disappear. Freeing your feeling is freeing your inner light.

Here is the terrific truth and the first step to breaking up with this habit hindering happiness. Our thoughts are based on emotions and emotions are not real—BAM, yes I said it! Emotions will lie to you; emotions live in your head. Feelings are real and they are safe in your heart. Feelings always tell you the truth— always! Even though you may not like their message and you may wish it were different, your feelings will be a pathway to freedom.

The idea for breaking up with this habit hindering our happiness is to more freely access our feelings. When we get in touch with our feelings, we can become more resilient and resourceful. We move through problems more gracefully, and we have more confidence in making once-difficult decisions. When we can tune in to our feelings, rather than our emotions, we can get honest with the situations in our lives and work through them more clearly. By getting in touch with your feelings, you have a set-point for climbing to new heights. If you free your feelings and recognize that you are feeling sad, this joy route teaches you to reach for a higher-level feeling, which will help you feel better. The Abraham-Hicks metaphysical teachings call this the Emotional Guidance Scale.

Abraham-Hicks developed a list of emotions that can help you work from feeling bad to feeling better in any situation. If you find what you are currently feeling on the scale, and then try to find thoughts that feel just a tad bit better, you have created a shift that can help you feel better in the moment. I call this baby steps toward joy, and I have found that it is the fastest way to lasting happiness. In one of my all-time favorite books, *Ask and it is Given* by Jerry and Esther Hicks, in chapter 22, the authors provide the feelings scale.

THE EMOTIONAL GUIDANCE SCALE

1. Joy/Appreciation/Empowered/Freedom/Love
2. Passion
3. Enthusiasm/Eagerness/Happiness
4. Positive Expectation/Belief
5. Optimism
6. Hopefulness
7. Contentment
8. Boredom
9. Pessimism
10. Frustration/Irritation/Impatience
11. "Overwhelment"
12. Disappointment
13. Doubt
14. Worry
15. Blame

16. Discouragement
17. Anger
18. Revenge
19. Hatred/Rage
20. Jealousy
21. Insecurity/Guilt/Unworthiness
22. Fear/Grief/Depression/Despair/Powerlessness

Notice that the feelings that are lower down on the emotional scale are more fearful and negative. If you tune in to your feelings and recognize that you are feeling fear, you can use this Emotional Guidance Scale to pull your way into a happier state. Looking at the scale, you will see that one feeling above fear is guilt. Reaching for the feelings within the next higher step can help you pull into a higher vibration emotion. The idea is to pull your way into the top layers of happiness, joy, and bliss. For example, with my client who used to suffer with overeating, she tried this method out and it looked something like this: "I just ate an entire bag of potato chips. I can't control myself; I am *powerless*. I am so bloated, gross, and fat. I *hate* myself and feel *guilty*. I am angry that I can't get it together. I *blame* myself for being so overweight, and I *worry* no one will love me for me."

When she came to me with this thought pattern, we identified the core emotions and where they were on the emotional guidance scale. If you look to the list, you will see each emotion has a high number by it. The higher the number, the lower the satisfaction level.

Powerlessness = 22

Hatred = 19

Guilt = 21

Anger = 17

Blame = 15

Worry = 14

After we looked at this, I asked her if she could pull herself into higher emotions. Could she move from worry to disappointment, then disappointment to frustration or content then to hopeful or appreciation? She was able to move one step at a time. She changed her outlook on her problem by paying attention to her feelings and pulling herself into a higher emotional state. You can do it too.

Try it out right now. Think about a situation that has been causing you stress, despair, or anxiety and free your feelings by asking yourself how you feel in this situation. Look at the Emotional Guidance Scale and see if you can access a higher-level vibrational feeling in reference to the situation. This is the joy route to happiness. Freeing our feelings can be fun when we give ourselves permission to feel them fully. Let's dive deeper.

AWESOME ACTION 1:
Identify Your Emotions vs. Feelings

The first step to joyfully bust this habit is to understand the true difference between your emotions (head) and feelings (heart). Both emotions and feelings can have an effect on your body and mind. Emotions affect you because they are rooted in some past experience and will try to rule your choices by reminding you of the consequences you suffered, the mistakes and failures of your past. When we listen to our emotions, we stay stuck in our past. Generated by the ego mind, they are most often triggered by current dilemmas that remind you of what happened in a similar experience in your past. Because they are often fear based and can contain other people's energy (remember the outward worldview reflected in them), emotions are very unreliable and self-limiting.

Let's try it out together.

1. Pick a troubling situation in your life. Ask what your thoughts around the situation are, and what is causing you the most stress.
2. Now drop to your heart and access your feelings about the situation. How do you feel about the situation in this moment?
3. Go on a jaunt to the Emotional Guidance Scale and focus on reaching for a higher-level feeling in this moment. The goal is to pull yourself into a higher, more positive emotional state. So pull your way up, one emotion at a time, to the next level higher up. Eventually you will reach a place of passion or joy.

Do you want to go even deeper? The following adventure for your soul can help you deep dive into this joy route. (This meditation is also available for video download; access details are at the end of the chapter.)

FREE YOUR FEELINGS MEDITATION

1. Think about a situation you are currently in and a decision you are trying to make about it. (Maybe you are starting a new business, changing careers, leaving a relationship, or thinking about having kids.)
   - Take a deep breath; breathe in and out three times softly and consciously. This will ground you and help center your thoughts so you can become aware of your feelings.
   - Be present, and forget about what will happen in the future; only focus on now. Pick one scenario to focus on first and ask, "If I do this, how does it feel?"

- Try to avoid thinking and just focus on feeling. You don't need to act on it, just be present.
- Breathe in and out, and continue to focus on the feeling. Does it feel expansive; do you feel uplifted and joyful? Or does it feel heavy, restricted, and fearful?

2. Now think of the situation and consider the opposite scenario. So if you were thinking of leaving your job, now consider staying at your job and feel your feelings.

- Do you feel an inward shift? Focus on this path and feel how it feels to you.

Which visualization made you feel more peaceful, expansive, happy, or relaxed?

Which choice made you feel tense, uneasy, or agitated?

Did you hold your breath when considering either thought?

The thought you felt more relaxed and at ease with is your true desire. That is your answer. Trust it.

Now be willing to receive guidance on how to step into this new reality. You don't have to have all the answers right now, but being able to access your feelings on the situation can help you align with your highest good and move forward with more grace and ease. For example, if it feels more freeing to leave your job, then trust that is a path for you, but you don't have to know the exact steps to take right now. They will be revealed to you through your feelings and gut instinct.

AWESOME ACTION 2: Free Your Feelings

One way to identify your feeling is to ask if it feels loving and real. Your inner voice will chime in to let you know the feeling is real; you may get a feeling, you may hear your inner voice, or you may even feel a knowing. These are all techniques your inner voice may use to let you know you are feeling rather than reacting with emotion.

Freeing your feelings takes practice, but asking objectively in each moment how you feel can help you access your heart center more easily. This will help you ensure your choices are aligned with your authentic feelings. Your heart is your compass and your inner guidance is your truth, not the emotions that are the results of outward situations. Trusting yourself means trusting your heart and freeing your feelings moment by moment.

Over the next thirty days, ask in every moment that feels stressful, "How do I feel?" and then reaffirm your choice by repeating these words:

"My choices are grounded in love. I align with my true feelings; it is safe to feel them fully."

☙

MOTIVATIONAL MANTRA

"I trust my heart.
It knows what my head has yet to figure out."

BONUS RESOURCE

If you want to take this step deeper, download this guided audio meditation:

"Free Your Feelings," from the *Adventures for Your Soul* meditation album. Available on iTunes, Amazon.com, or playwiththeworld.com/home/shop/

FOUR

Play Truth or Dare with Your Inner Child

HABIT HINDERING HAPPINESS
Our dreams don't intimidate us.

Let's go back in time and visit mini-you. This is the you before "adulting," before you became a responsible, stressed, eager-to-please, overworked, underjoyed, dreams-on-the-back-burner adult. This is "adulting": sacrificing your desires for the demands, responsibilities, and expectations that come with being an adult.

No matter what your childhood was like, we can all look back to a moment in our life when we were young, happy, and free. We had dreams of becoming astronauts, world-famous singers, or, if you were like me, a mermaid. We think growing up is full of magic, full of inspiration, sprinkled with glitter and love. Visit a time in your childhood where you felt this effortless magic of life and the freedom to be you. You felt safe and secure, and there were no demands or pressures on who or what you were. You were able to dream. What did you dream about? Try for a moment to revisit the little you and see how happy you are. What are you doing?

This is your true essence. This is what you value. Getting in touch with younger selves allows us to get to the heart of our true desires.

But sometime after that perfect moment, things change . . . BAM! Life happens. Mom and Dad get a divorce, we see death, sickness, traumas, turbulent times mangled with depression, addictions, fear, hate, and crime. Ugh! Life becomes an uphill struggle. We start to let go of our dreams because life demands so much from us. We put more faith in our fear because the world teaches us to expect the worst; planning for miracles is for the disillusioned or the enchanted wanderlusters, frivolously frolicking about with their heads stuck in the clouds. Those people, the adults who still have dreams, are disillusioned; don't they know that dreaming will set them up to fail? Don't the dreamers know that following your heart hurts? It is much safer to stay unhappy and stuck than it is to give ourselves permission to play with the world and desire more for ourselves. At least this seems to be the mentality for so many as we age.

Our mothers and fathers, grandparents, friends, teachers, and even neighbors have all told us that dreaming is for the unrealistic; playing big in life is scary, and sticking to the status quo will help you become successful. Realize that people who urge you to be realistic generally want you to accept their version of reality. They think that you will be happy if you follow the plan set forth by so many. It is a strategic plan to attain security, success, and predictability. Go to school, get a job, fall in love, get married, pop out cute little chubby babies, then retire with enough money to travel, and finally, sit on the porch and reflect on the good life. This works for many, but for most, at one point or another, we fall into despair. Maybe the children grow up and leave for college and we are forced to look at who we are without them. Or perhaps the person you said "I do" to is suddenly saying "not you." Or maybe we get laid off from the career we spent the past twenty years devoting our life to. At each transition we are paralyzed by the big unknown and we are forced to ask ourselves "What now?" Who we thought we were is gone, and now we need to choose a new path.

The truth is, these crossroads, as difficult as the circumstances may be, can actually be blessings or pathways. When situations such as divorce, layoff, even death or sickness arise, we are caught in between who we thought we were and who we really are. It can be an opportunity to tap into our long-forgotten dreams and get back to our true selves. For those of us who left our little dreamer back in childhood, the process of dreaming has been forgotten. And if we had given ourselves permission to set goals and dream, the goals we set are the ones that can be managed with little maintenance or perspiration. For many people, dreams are things of childhood memories, possibly to be allowed to show up again at retirement.

Before leaving my corporate job and waking up to the work I do today, I too had forgotten how to dream.

Let's go back in time several years to my own experience in the corporate world. This is an excerpt from my first published story, which was featured in *Chicken Soup for the Soul: Find Your Happiness:*

My coworker who sat behind me was getting married. He proudly pushed down the taped corners of his engagement photo on his cubicle wall. He looked over at me and observed, "Did you ever notice that what people put up in their office space is a reflection of what they care most about?" I took a quick mental snapshot of the office and realized that my cubicle was the only one not overstuffed with chubby-baby photos and cherished significant others. In fact, I didn't have any family photos on display. My show-and-tell was a flooded collage of postcards from cities I longed to go to and places I had already experienced. Puzzled by this, I asked him what my area said about me. He matter-of-factly responded, "You want to escape."

His words felt like lightning striking my chest. How was it that a work acquaintance knew me better than I knew myself? I'm not sure why I ignored that blazing red flag, but at the time I was in the business of missing the obvious. Why would I want to escape? I had carefully crafted every aspect of my current life, from the city I lived in to the company that I worked for. I had actively pursued this career in advertising. I had put myself in a graphic design program after college, and had graduated at the top of my class, all in an eager effort to live the dream. I was determined to work in a big advertising agency, and live in a fast-paced city. And here I was!

I didn't know that the majority of people in the world didn't cry themselves to sleep at night. My tears even crept into my workplace. I thought it was normal to cry in the bathroom. I violently pushed forward, ignoring my inner voice, completely blind to my true purpose. I never once stopped to think about the other red flags. The fact that I had lived in five different cities in a span of three years didn't seem odd to me. The reality that everyone I knew was collecting wedding registry lists and picking out house paint swatches, while I was more excited to collect more passport stamps. It never dawned on me that my true purpose was to play with the world. The truth was that I had become pretty good at being someone else. I had, unbeknownst to me, convinced myself and every single person that I knew that I was capable and more than willing to climb the corporate ladder. The rest of the world was falling in love, planning weddings, and breeding that love into little babies. Meanwhile, I was lost, alone, and loveless.

I figured there might be something to this love thing; I should give it a try. I finally got up enough nerve to ask myself out on a date. The first encounter was simple; I took myself to coffee and brought along my laptop. Within seconds of typing my first sentence, I was attached. Like any transformational love affair, I quickly wanted to spend every waking moment together. I hadn't taken any sick days or vacation in over four years. All of a sudden I was calling in sick so I could spend the entire day soaked up in my writing. It was as if I was in a secret love affair with my true self, and cheating on my professional career. It felt illicit, but I couldn't deny how natural and comfortable this new relationship felt. Even though I was sneaking behind my day job's back, the real deception was with my position in advertising. That was the relationship that was a false reality.

This infatuation with writing grew rapidly into an appreciation and dedication to me; it was an unconditional love because I had found my true purpose. It was time to declare my love to the world, so I took my writing on a honeymoon. We arrived in the most romantic city in the world . . . Bonjour, Paris, France! I spent two weeks saturated in the experience of Paris, a time filled with exploration, amazement, and awe. On a whim I sent in some of my travel blogs to editors and book publishers. A few months later I received a letter from an editor that informed me that my story had been selected to appear in an upcoming book. Before I could finish reading the letter, my knees collapsed as I fell to the floor; for the first time in my entire life, tears of extraordinary happiness gushed from my eyes. I was going to be a published author. I didn't know that this was a dream of mine until my heart sang out. Until this point, I had pretended to be someone I was not; it had proved to be loveless and unfulfilling. I knew what I had to do; it was time for me to break up with advertising.

Like any involved relationship, I got scared. Fear crept in and cuddled up next to me. I worried about finding money to pay my bills, and where I would live as a travel writer. Real-life issues set in, and my dreams went back to just being a "wouldn't it be nice?" idea. My ego spit on the fantasy and condescendingly stated, "Who are you to gallivant around the world?" So I stayed miserable and depressed. That is, of course, until the Universe had finally had enough of me hiding out from my own shadow. Finally the bubble exploded and I was laid off from my job. I was too stubborn to see the signs before then, but this was the Universe's way of ripping the blindfold off. It was my divine intervention; it was the miracle that saved my life. I received a healthy severance that gave me the confidence to move myself toward my new purpose, to launch my new career, and to inspire people to play with the world.

I share this story because it demonstrates my disenchantment with life and how I had forgotten how to dream. I forgot to put myself into my own life. I was going through the motions, but feeling a void with every action. I was not alone. It is a human tendency to do this, because we are conditioned to fall into these behaviors. The world tells us what will make us happy, and yet we walk around feeling disconnected, alone, and unsupported, not because we aren't trying, but because we aren't dreaming. I had forgotten how to dream, and though I did everything I was supposed to do—went to the fancy school, met a man who wanted to marry me, landed a great career with a great salary and health benefits—at the end of it all, I was still unhappy. I had forgotten how to dream, and it wasn't until I started to dream bigger that my world changed. I was able to turn my personal pain into hope.

If you are in a place in your life where you feel stuck or where things feel chaotic, realize that you don't have to be a victim of your circumstances. Allowing yourself to go inward and play truth or dare with your inner child will help you break up the monotony and fall fully in love with your life.

JOY ROUTE
Play truth or dare with your Inner child.

The path of least resistance is the journey into the heart. The little you, the one that was left behind when your parents both worked late jobs, the little you that was picked on by classmates or felt unsupported in your dreams, the little you that was told, "that will never work," that you would not be able to do what you love, the little you still stuck, paralyzed by the naysayers, is longing for a hug.

Visit mini-you and give yourself a huge hug. Let your inner child know that you are here and ready to put those "mini-you dreams" into action. Most of us have inner children that long to be heard, but we suffocate their desires with "adulting" demands. We fail to ask ourselves what we really want. We don't have clarity, so we don't have desires. We have conditioned ourselves to seek out what we are told we should want, but when something happens like a layoff or disease, the rug is pulled out from under us, and we are sent in a new direction.

Instead of suffocating our dreamer or waiting for life to unfold before we pursue our dreams, the fastest way to happiness is to dream bigger, and to dream bigger right now. Don't worry about the state your life is currently in; your dreams matter now, and the little you is empowered and needs you to believe in those dreams. This joy route focuses on playing truth or dare with your inner child because most of us don't know what we want. If I were to ask you what your biggest dream is right now, could you answer me? Most people can't! They get that "Bambi stuck in headlights" look. This is because we have grown so out of touch with our inner child by the status quo of "adulting" that we have forgotten how to play. That's right, we forget how to do one of the most natural and joyful things: to play. When is the last time you played? I don't mean just reading a book for fun or having coffee with a friend. Those are adult playtimes. I mean a child's playtime, the raw feeling of living life fully—think sidewalk chalk, hopscotch, skipping down the street, running as fast as you can on the beach until you burst out with tears of laughter, squeezing your dog so tightly that she licks you all over. When did you last experience in-the-moment, fully present, completely captivating playtime? Children are so happy because they access this part of themselves daily, moment by moment. Just think of the joy little babies bring to our lives— they, themselves, are bursting with joy, and everything is an adventure, everything is a game. As we grow old we lose this sense of wonder, but to access your fullest potential, letting yourself be childish, is part of the happiness plan. When you think of yourself as a child, there are certain clues that can lead you to dream bigger. Embrace your inner child!

AWESOME ACTION 1:
Play Truth or Dare with Your Inner Child

Have you ever played the game truth or dare? It is a game many children play to help them learn more about each other. Your friends ask you "truth" or "dare?" If you answer "truth," you must tell the truth no matter what the question is. But if you answer "dare," no matter what you are asked to do, you must happily accept the challenge. The fastest way to get out of the crippling monotony of "adulting" is to play truth or dare with your inner child. Let's try it out!

How do you fall in love with your life? You invite your inner child along for the ride. You get curious and ask interesting questions of your inner child, ones that can help you reveal your truth.

You dare yourself to try new things, to pursue experiences you've always wanted to explore. You trust your instincts and arrive fully in each moment—present, focused, and in awe.

Pull out your joy journal and answer these key questions below.

TRUTH:
Get really honest with yourself and answer these key questions from the perspective of your inner child.

1. What did I love to do as a child?
2. When was I happiest as a child?
3. As a child, what did I want to be when I grew up?
4. What five qualities did I express the most as a child?

DARE:
Dare yourself to try new situations.

What is something you've always wanted to do, but were too scared to go for it? Think from your heart and let your inner desires come to the surface. Dare yourself to try it.

After you answer the truth questions, you will have more clarity. Dare yourself to try something you have always wanted to do—skydiving, cooking class, learning French, traveling to Peru—whatever it is, pursue your heart's desire. Dream bigger and let your inner child play. All of this magic can start in your mind. Your imagination is your golden ticket to happiness. If you can visualize it first, it can become a reality. If you don't allow yourself to play in your mind and explore new ideas, you will be stuck in "adulting." This joy route is about having fun, and literally going out to recess.

For the next thirty days, dare yourself to dream bigger. Each day it will become more comfortable; as you take action toward each dare, you will strengthen your trust muscles, which in turn will build your confidence. You will see that booking a one-way ticket to Hawaii isn't that odd after all, or that pitching your book idea to a literary agent isn't as wild as you once imagined. Your dreams will become crystal clear, and you will have the courage to follow through on them. Have fun daring yourself to dream bigger.

Once you put this joy route into action, you will feel more alive, passionate, and purpose filled. The dream in your heart will pop out daily, and you will feel more inner peace because you are aligned with your true self.

After you get into the habit of playing truth or dare with your inner child, you can translate your dreams into a plan in chapter 16, Be a Goal Digger. That chapter will help you blueprint your dreams so they will become effortless and fun to achieve. Have fun dreaming bigger and reaching for the stars. Your inner child is ready to come out and play.

MOTIVATIONAL MANTRA

"I'm inspired by my courageous heart.
I listen to its guidance daily."

FIVE

Allow Awareness

We get comfortable being uncomfortable.

The heart of the idea to write this book was inspired by this particular emotional habit, of getting comfortable being uncomfortable. The idea came to me when I recognized the patterns I used to fall into before coming to the work I do today. For the majority of my life, I had stayed in situations and repeated patterns because it was what I was used to, and being uncomfortable was the safe route. Being uncomfortable—whether it was in an overweight body and hating the way I felt in my own skin, staying in a job that I disliked, or dating men who I knew were wrong for my big picture—soon became comfortable. Being uncomfortable is slightly comfortable because it keeps us in our comfort zone. It is safe. It is expected. It is normal.

The safe and predictable route is comfortable because we feel safe, we feel protected, and we feel as if we have control of our lives. If we have a little extra layer on our bodies because it makes us feel safe, or we stay in a job we really don't like for the security of a paycheck, or we stay in a relationship because it is easier than leaving, we have succumbed to letting the uncomfortable become our new comfortable.

Pushing out of our comfort zone and reaching for that healthy body, reaching for that dream job, or choosing to be single and independent rather than leaning on a relationship that does not serve us can be scary. Although it is scary, my life today is proof that it is worth it. On the other side of being uncomfortable are joy, peace, and abundant love.

Why is being uncomfortable the norm for so many of us? As we talked about in chapter 1, everything we do is based on a reward system. Every action has result, and when the result is rewarding, we will continue to choose that action. Now, you may ask, why do we choose things that are ultimately not rewarding? Why do we eat that second piece of chocolate cake when we know that we'll eventually see an unwanted number on the scale and it could adversely affect our health? Why do we get entangled with that bad boy we know will eventually break our heart? Why do we stay in a job that we know is a dead end and will lead nowhere? It's because in the reward system, we don't differentiate between immediate gratification and long-term benefit. That chocolate cake is so comforting now, Mr. Bad Boy is so exciting, and that dead-end job pays the bills. It's what feels good now. The problem is that the more we choose a particular reward, the more our brain and body become accustomed to it. It becomes habitual. So even when the action stops being rewarding, we continue with the pattern. Our brain and body adapt to this new normal, and we're comfortable with the uncomfortable. After all, we have spent most of our life settling, or believing that this is the best option we can get, and we have no real motive to push toward a happier state of being.

This habit hindering happiness is very common for many people I work with, and it was a big one for me when I started to write this book. We sometimes fall into hopeless thought patterns that become our safety net. Many women I work with in individual coaching sessions express their regret with their earlier years. Some are divorced and explain that they got married young because it was what they were "supposed to do" and it felt safe and comfortable. Years later, after they divorced, they have had time to reflect and see that perhaps their motivation for marriage was that they felt comfortable being slightly uncomfortable. Although they loved their husbands at the time, they stayed in an unhappy marriage, a marriage that made them uncomfortable, but it was actually comfortable because that is what was expected of them.

I see this pattern play out in romantic relationships for so many people. But it is not just with romantic love. It can be in any area of our lives.

My lifelong relationship with my body is my biggest example of getting comfortable being uncomfortable. No matter what shape or size I am or have been, whether thirty pounds underweight or fifty pounds overweight, or anything in between, I have always felt uncomfortable with my physical body.

I spent years studying my relationship to my own body and myself. The reality is that I always felt uncomfortable in my own skin. I couldn't look in the mirror, whether I was fat or thin, and I never believed people when they gave me compliments. My deep-rooted insecurity about my own body stemmed from my childhood. I traced this back to wanting to fit in. My family moved a lot when I was growing up, so I never had real roots. Each new school brought new bullies and new chances for me to strive to do everything I could to fit in, but striving for perfection caused me to cycle through bulimic and anorexic phases. I was quite literally starving for attention, and in the process starving my body to exhaustion. When that didn't work, when people still poked fun at me, I turned to food and gained weight. Being the largest girl in school certainly gave people more to pick on. I never felt like I fit in, nor did I feel accepted. I would take this pain out on my body. I blamed my physical body for all of my problems. I would look in the mirror and squeeze my face so hard my skin would pulse with pain. If only I could scrub this fat off. If only my body were normal, my life would be better. I spent decades fighting with myself, yelling at my body, abusing it physically, emotionally, and putting it in danger, all to try to fit in and be accepted. It wasn't until I started writing this book and practicing the actions I'm sharing with you that things began to shift for me.

I slowly began to realize that spending years uncomfortable in my body was more comfortable than accepting myself. Accepting myself meant really looking at where I was in my life and why I was there. Accepting myself meant getting real and facing some scary truths. Accepting myself meant feeling the pain that I had long tried to mask with obsessing over food and hating my body.

In order to become truly comfortable and never allow ourselves to settle into an uncomfortable state, we have to be honest with ourselves and face head-on our fat bodies, our low bank accounts, our toxic relationships, our unfulfilling jobs—and in spite of all this, love ourselves. It always comes back to our relationship with our self. Always. I finally accepted that for me it wasn't the excess weight on my hips or the number on the scale or the plus-size clothes, it was my relationship to myself. No matter what size I was, I never, ever liked myself. And in order to be truly comfortable, we have to love ourselves, we have to respect ourselves, and we have to believe we are worthy of our desires.

My epiphany came when I sat down and wrote a letter to my future self. This was after a food binge-fest and a thirty-minute episode of crying on the floor because I was bored and living an unmotivated life. At the time I was fifty pounds overweight, I was extremely frustrated and angry that things in my career were not going as smoothly as I wanted, and I was mad because I was single, which, in my mind, also meant unlovable.

In order to clear out all the garbage in my mind, I had to take a little mental trip to see my future self—the one who has a balanced relationship with food, the one who is fulfilled with every moment of life and each experience; the future me, the one who has a book deal and is spreading her message to millions, and the one who has extraordinary self-love. That girl felt foreign to me. After all, I had just shoved two pints of Ben & Jerry's down my throat trying to feel something, anything, to escape the numbing pain of my static life. I knew what my future self was like: She was truly happy, healthy, and in love with life. "I want to be her," I thought to myself. "I want to meet her." So I sat down and wrote to her.

Dear Future Me,

I see you smiling, sitting so peacefully and in awe. You are looking at me, your younger more naïve, more determined, more self-righteous self, and you have nothing but love and gratitude for me. You watch me cry on my living room floor, completely bored and unmotivated by life, depressed at how large my body has become. You see me struggle daily. You see the pain I carry around in my heart and you watch me avoid mirrors because I hate what I see in the mirror. You see me have momentary outbursts and cry with furious fits of rage.

But you also see that I make it through. You see that I am okay. My pain, my struggles, my issues are not what define me. You see that I make it through this rough patch and you know that I come out stronger, smarter, and more aware than ever before.

Future me, you are so elegant and poised, with a sophisticated, laid-back manner that makes me want to get to know you much sooner. I see you smile with gratitude for all of the lessons I am in the thick of. The gut-wrenching painful moments of extreme self-hate, followed by harsh words and flurries of condescending tones, and you are proud to have them be a way of your past. You made it through fully and hold nothing but positive, loving thoughts for yourself. You love yourself so much it shines through every pore of your body. Your energy is light and tender; I want to get to know you sooner.

Future me, your light shines breathlessly and your energy and love are infectious. You have a knowing about you that is wise, patient, and graceful. You see that everything is always in right order and what I am going through is part of my bigger plan. It is as if you know that all of this turbulent stress was divinely put into my life to help me become the person I need to be.

Your eyes are soft and full of love for everything. I see that you have compassion that beams through your pores. You have so much love to give the world, and you are shining it at every moment.

Future self, I see you and you are so proud of me, for learning these lessons, for rolling up my sleeves and doing the work on myself and getting into the trenches of my own life to prepare me for my next chapter. You are oozing with awareness and you see that I am getting it. Day by day, I am learning.

I choose to work toward you, and by taking responsibility for my life, you are able to be you. You smile because you see that I get it, that the choices I make today affect you and your daily life in the future. You see that I am showing up and doing the best I can. And what may feel like not enough or a failure to me is more than enough in your eyes. You are proud and honored to be me.

You have become everything you knew you could because of what I am experiencing right now. This pain, this troubled heart, the burdens of my yesterdays are slowly being released. Day by day I choose to show up and do the work on myself to be the person you have become.

Future self, you show me what is possible. You shine love and self-respect in a manner that I can't grasp in this moment, but I am trying, and you tell me that is enough. I am so thankful that you take care of yourself every single day. You love yourself both in and out and you don't need anyone's approval. I am so honored to become you. Future self, the most powerful thing you are showing me is what is possible with our life. I can't wait to meet you.

You have let go of worrying about any outcome; you know that everything always works out. You have forgiven your ex-lovers and fallen in love with yourself fully.

You are not defined by your problems or any situation that comes to you. You ride the waves of life with such ease that it makes me want to catch up to you faster.

Future self, I want to be where you are, happy, healthy, free of worries, in love with every part of my life. I see that together we figure it out. I know that my life is a moment-by-moment web of intricate experiences and reactions that help me shape you. I am working to make myself better for you, for us.

I am showing up for all of my assignments. I am choosing to be happy. And I am choosing to love openly and honestly. Future self, I am going to take big risks because I know you know I need to. I am not going to settle EVER AGAIN.

I am going to leap into the unknown and follow my heart fully. I am going to become the person you know I can be. Future self, you are my guide and you show me what is possible for our life. You show me that no matter what life throws at us, we are stronger, smarter, and healthier and more beautiful than ever, not because we rise above it, even though we do, but because we have the courage to keep going.

Our experiences make us who we are. I choose to let my dreams and successes define me; I release my problems and my attachment to identifying with them. I am no longer weighed down by self-loathing thoughts. I choose to be happy.

Future self, you rock and I am so unbelievably proud I get to become you.

Love forever,
Younger, not so together, sad
and overweight,
doing the best she can,
Shannon

This letter became my path to emotional joy. I allowed myself to see that it all works out. I can be happy and I can choose joy, and I do not have to wait until my future. This letter became the catalyst to breaking this habit hindering happiness. No longer could I allow myself to stay in an uncomfortable situation knowing that my future self is rooting for me.

Many of us have spent so many years being uncomfortable that it has become comfortable. We're so comfortable being uncomfortable that being healthy, happy, or debt free is initially an uncomfortable state, and we quickly fall back into the constricting state of being uncomfortable. When we have a glimpse of a better way to be, when we see our healthy, vibrant, leaner body, or where we are living our dream job, or in a relationship that lifts us up and doesn't brings us down, we start to take steps toward that better way. But as I said earlier, every action has an outcome. And inevitably, when you start making changes, things start to shift. Maybe life circumstances seem to get more chaotic, and so it seems much easier to fall back than to push forward into the great big sea of the unknown. The unknown is terribly scary, and if we have spent most of our life in a state of settling, it is more comfortable to us than branching out into a world where we don't know what to expect.

Or perhaps you start walking toward your true self and others react negatively. I know from personal experience that every time I've tried to move toward something new and better for my life, people have had strong reactions. Changing the status quo makes other people nervous. If what we all want is to be loved and accepted, and we start showing pieces of the REAL us to others, and they react negatively, we shy away from our true self. Most of the time the guilt creeps in—guilt for making others uncomfortable, guilt for rocking the boat, guilt for even believing we could be anything but what we already are.

What is really happening? When we choose to be comfortable being uncomfortable, we are actually cheating on our true self with a false ego version of us. The ego mind-set is based on fear, and fear will always try to push us into what feels safe. This is why we stay in jobs we hate, this is why we stay in relationships that are toxic, why we spend all our money, overeat or starve ourselves, why we bury our dreams under a rock. The truth is, we are all terrified of being our true self, because what if our true self isn't accepted? There may have been a moment in your life where you showed a piece of your true self—maybe you told your parents you wanted to change careers or move to a new city, or maybe you told your significant other you want to go back to school—and the reaction was less than stellar from your support posse. What happens then? We train ourselves to shy away from our desires, we decide in that moment that being accepted and feeling loved is better than following our heart.

But we see that this is not working. It creates a constant internal struggle, and for me it led to emotional abuse, drug addictions, clinical depression, an obese body, as well as extreme lack of self-love and confidence. It wasn't until I truly started to give myself permission to tap into my heart's real desires that things began to shift.

It is possible to live a life that you are 100 percent comfortable with. Imagine your relationships being honest, pure, and full of integrity, you are living in a location you feel passionate about, you get to do what you love daily, and you have more money than you know what to do with. Getting truly comfortable means you unapologetically stand behind your own self. In order to choose this path we must first allow awareness.

⌒〰

JOY ROUTE
Allow awareness.

We always have a choice in life, and choosing to put yourself first is a choice. It means that you are able to access the piece of yourself, buried deep inside, that wants to show the world who you really are. Here is the beautiful little secret about this emotional habit: the real you, the one that you have hidden inside for fear of being unloved and unaccepted, has a place in this world. The real you belongs. The real you is supposed to be here and is supposed to show your true colors. The more you show your real self, the more you shed your layers of discomfort, the more the world can reflect your true essence. From my own personal experience, once I started to stand up for my true desires and treat my body with respect, I realized that what other people think of me doesn't really have anything to do with me. I started to unapologetically honor myself. This meant trusting my heart's pull and giving myself permission to be who I really was. As I did this, the drug addictions stopped, my extra emotional and physical weight returned to balance, the relationships that were not really right for me disappeared from my life. The more I showed my real self, the more love I felt from the world. Most importantly, I realized that real deep love and acceptance in life is not about other people; it can only come from within.

As you step into your true essence, you will be rewarded in grand ways. You will also find that the universe will grant you more opportunities. The more you allow yourself to express your true self, the more comfortable you are. Whatever your true heart's desire is, you owe it to YOURSELF and the world to be you. The world does not need you to hide your true self in an effort to fit in. Guess what, you already fit. The world loves you as you are. And as you allow yourself to show your true colors, you will see the world as a safe place; you will see that it is comfortable and more loving than you ever thought possible.

The real magic happens when you trust that your heart is your greatest guide; that pull that has been nagging at you for some time is the real you. That pull is you leading you gently to REAL lasting happiness. This uncomfortable state that you have called living, the one that is filled with guilt, can be a portal to your true self.

The more I stepped into my true self, and the more comfortable I was, people who no longer fit in my life fell away. Once I really stepped into my true self, my life changed for the better. My relationships are now much more rewarding, and I am surrounded by uplifting people who support my heart's goals. I was able to trust my future self and allow my heart to become my own best friend. This led me to be an abundant travel writer, speaker, bestselling author, life coach, and lover of life. When your heart is your own best friend, you don't need acceptance from those around you, because you recognize that you are already accepted. When you love yourself, you fit in. To truly live an extraordinary life, you must trust that you are enough as you are. You do not need to try to be someone you are not; stop letting yourself be uncomfortable and stand up for yourself. You matter and you belong. In order to truly break the emotional habit of getting comfortable being uncomfortable, we have to first allow awareness.

The joy route is an adventure into your own current reality. Just like my letter to my future self stated, I had to accept and get honest about where I was to get to where I wanted to go.

Allowing awareness is all about self-compassion. In order to move through this emotional habit and release it for good, we must sign a pact that we will be kind, loving, and gentle to ourselves through the transition. Transitions can be scary, and you will find that the more you resist them, the more turbulent they will seem to be.

Turbulence feels like a jolt to our normal routine, and it can be disturbing. In fact, it can be downright scary, as your mind creates a scenario for the new situation that is filled with danger. It's a lot like turbulence on a plane trip. How many times have you flown on an airplane and had a turbulent ride? You're flying along comfortably and all of a sudden a bump, a dip, a drop jolts you out of your comfort zone. It's likely that you felt fear, and as the turbulence continued, you moved on to panic, which created a scenario where your plane was going to crash. You sit up a little straighter in your seat, tighten your seat belt, and pray to God as you grasp your armrest. The same thing happens in life; we are cruising along a standard route, but choose to go down a different path, deciding to start being healthier, to leave our relationship, or go back to school. We may announce it to another person or we may decide to take a step toward that new desire, and BOOM!—turbulence. Our mind instantly moves to fear and paints a devastating outcome resulting in angry lovers, parents, and friends, and disastrous consequences.

What I found out from talking to pilots is that turbulence is literally nothing. Pilots don't worry about turbulence at all. In fact, one pilot told me it is like your car going over a speed bump. When was the last time you drove your car over a speed bump and you started freaking out that you might die? It doesn't happen, because we recognize speed bumps are just a caution to slow down. Well, the way I see it, the resistance we feel in our life when we start to step into a new path is a lot like a speed bump; it is just a signal to remind you to proceed slowly, but also a sign that you are on the right path and that things are not as bad as you think they are. The turbulence you feel at first from trusting yourself and moving forward is nothing more than a speed bump to guide you into your new life.

When you truly allow awareness for this process, you will never want to go back to being uncomfortable. You have a place in this world, and the more real you can be, the more love you will feel.

Now let's put this into action. As I said before, trusting your own heart and letting it be your guide will be the adventure that will guide you to lasting happiness.

AWESOME ACTION 1: Recognize Resistance

Where in your life have you been resisting your heart's pull? You can usually tell by looking at the area of your life where you feel the most uncomfortable, and yet comfortable because it has been that way for so long. Maybe you are uncomfortable in your body, and you resist taking healthy steps and improving your diet because people around you make fun of you for trying a new diet. Maybe you have tried in the past, but nothing has worked. Whatever area of your life feels heavy and uncomfortable, focus on that for this exercise. To break this emotional habit, look at the resistance and ask yourself, "What am I afraid of?" Feel free to pull out your joy journal and freewrite on this idea. It will help you dive deeper to sit with it for a moment. Usually there is a contrast between the place you are in your life and where you want to be. The resistance pops up because you see where you want to be, and it does not align with where you currently are. Give yourself time to write about this topic.

Now write out what areas are most uncomfortable for you.

AWESOME ACTION 2: Trust Your Heart's Pull

In the situation where you feel the most resistance, the one you feel most uncomfortable in, dig a little deeper and ask what your heart has been suggesting about the situation. Again, you can open up your joy journal and write this out.

My heart is guiding me to . . .

Once you make a list of your heart's true desires, you can start believing in these ideas.

AWESOME ACTION 3: Allow Awareness

Allowing awareness is the process of uncovering your heart's true desires. Your heart is your best friend, and when you allow it to be your confidante in life, you will never have to feel uncomfortable again. The more you let yourself be the real you, the more love you will feel. The love we settle for before tapping into allowing awareness can feel like real love, but anything grounded in uncomfortable emotions is actually fear based. Let your motivation be love instead of fear. Allow awareness for the entire process. The notion of allowing awareness can be your guiding mantra as you move forward. In any situation where you find yourself feeling uncomfortable, you can pause for a moment and repeat in your mind, "I allow awareness for this process to unfold." This means you must drop from your head into your heart. This means you must be in the moment; moment by moment, give yourself permission to be authentic to your true self. Follow your heart's pull and trust that it is guiding you toward your true destiny.

One of my private coaching clients has a health blog. She expressed that she loved sharing healthy tips with people, but she often felt like a fraud. She felt like she would have days where she didn't feel healthy, and she would be writing but feeling uncomfortable about what she was saying. I suggested that she practice being true to herself, and sharing the downs as well as the ups. She gave herself permission to share her personal experiences more openly and with authentic honesty. The next week I spoke to her, and she happily exclaimed that she had written a blog post on her health site about how she was feeling unhealthy. With that vulnerable posting, she had more comments and shares than ever before. This is a perfect reminder that the more authentic you are to yourself, the more the world can respond. In your own life, think about where you can be more vulnerable and express your truth. Give this idea time, but realize that allowing awareness means compassionately dropping from your head into your heart. Let your heart be your compass; it will guide you to live every day of your life feeling comfortable being comfortable.

AWESOME ACTION 4: Dear Future Me

Now is the pivotal moment for you to break through this habit hindering happiness. Writing a letter to your future self can be a true gift. Your journey will unfold more gracefully when you are aware of and aligning your current path with your future self, the one who has overcome the tough times you currently face, the future you who is happy and healthy. Visit that version of you. You can do a mental exercise using my downloadable audio meditation "Go on a Future Field Trip," or simply write out a letter to yourself. Be kind, but be honest. Give your future self the benefit of the doubt that she or he has risen to new heights because of your current situation. This can be empowering, and the letter can help motivate you to action.

∞

MOTIVATIONAL MANTRA

"I am willing to express my authentic self with courage and compassion. It is safe to be me."

BONUS RESOURCES

If you want to take this step deeper, download these guided audio meditations:

"Allow Awareness," from the *Adventures for Your Soul* meditation album. Available on iTunes, Amazon.com, or playwiththeworld.com/home/shop/

"Future Field Trip," from the *Adventures for Your Soul* meditation album. Available on iTunes, Amazon.com, or playwiththeworld.com/home/shop/

SIX

Me Matters

We think self-love is selfish.

My friend and branding client Rhonda Britten, founder of the Fearless Living Institute, bestselling author, and Emmy Award winner, says there are two types of people in this world: those who blame everyone else for their problems, and those who blame themselves. Do you blame others for the situations gone awry in your life? Or do you internalize your pain and self-sabotage yourself in punishment? Throughout my own life, I have always taken my pain and internalized it. For years, I would blame myself for not being good enough, not making my relationships work, staying in situations long past their expiration date—this included jobs, men, and homes. No matter what was wrong with my life, it was always my fault. I would attract men who blamed the world for their issues, and of course, I thought I was their favorite scapegoat. Nothing was ever their fault, so it must be me. There was nothing I could do to make things better, so I must be to blame.

Maybe you can relate. What are the qualities of your relationships? Do you take on other people's issues and pain, or do you blame them for your own situations? I've worked with hundreds of people from all different walks of life, from celebrities to regular people just trying to make it by, and what I found was the amount of love you have for yourself is indirectly proportionate to the amount of blame you will allow in your life. I know in my own experience, I was always blaming myself because I didn't love myself. I didn't value myself and I felt as if everything was my fault. Every man I dated, and even my closest girlfriends at the time, blamed the world for their problems, so I was the perfect partner for them. We were cozy cocreators, both reinforcing our own beliefs. We each played into one another's belief system like it was our full-time job. Because I didn't love myself and we both blamed me for everything, I was always consumed with guilt and focused on making things "right." I did everything I could to please them, in the process losing more of myself every day.

Putting my own needs first was not a daily practice. And when I did venture to comfort myself—some small act or token to make myself feel better or even self-care—I would eventually beat myself up. I blamed myself for sleeping in too late, eating too much ice cream, not saving enough money. Everything was always my fault . . . until one day it wasn't. I made the shift! This shift is putting yourself first; the shift is knowing that self-love is not selfish. The shift for me was, "Enough excuses, I want results."

The shift is something we all want when we come to work like this. The moment of BAM! Everything clicks and you are ready to release what no longer serves you, the moment you are ready to allow yourself to be happy, the moment you realize it is time to stop blaming and complaining and start acting in line with your desires. The shift is nothing shy of creative magic executed with honest intention. The shift is not an overnight experience; everything from the books we've read, the music we've listened to, the daily intentions, affirmations, positive thinking, and courses we've taken come together and BAM! We ignite an inner light that is so powerful and we can't go back. The shift is you declaring you are worth it!

The shift will not happen before you are ready. This is why we return to the familiar habits. We may try to break the addictions, or leave the toxic relationship, or walk away from the job we hate, but we return, and suffer in solitude because we keep ignoring our inner light. Why do we sacrifice our self and return to what no longer serves us? For most of us, it's because we believe that self-love is selfish. Being selfish and stepping forward into the job we really want, into the lifestyle we truly long for, or in the relationship we really deserve, could create a backlash of hate, fights, pain, and lonely roads ahead. So we suffocate our inner desires and play it safe in relationships, jobs, and situations that do not ignite our soul. And to cover up the inner turmoil, we resort to blame. Blaming others or ourselves conveniently masks our inner cries to be more, have more, and do more with our life.

Blame is a cousin of fear. Fear keeps us from falling in love with our life; it keeps us playing small and avoiding risk to protect what we have created. At night, blame cuddles up in our sheets as we lie awake wondering, "Is this all there is? Why am I not happy? Why am I alone? Why am I not where I want to be? Why do I hate myself?"

The shift can only happen when we let go of trying to please others and focus on pleasing ourselves, when we focus on our own heart's desires and choose self-love. For me the shift occurred when I could drop into my heart and sincerely say, "I am worth it, I matter."

Once you experience the shift, your old behaviors fall away naturally, but as I said, it doesn't happen overnight. It's kind of like learning a new language. At first you may struggle and stumble, working hard to make sense of what is foreign to you. But slowly you start to digest it, day by day, and with consistent, persistent effort, one day, you find you are able to hold an entire conversation with someone in the new language without any hiccups or hesitations. BAM! The shift.

In my personal coaching sessions, clients often ask, "When am I going to feel different? When am I going to see results?" My answer is always the same: when you stop expecting it to happen. Like learning a new language, falling in love with yourself will happen when you practice it daily. The results you seek come when practice collides with dedication and consistency.

By looking to something we want outside of ourselves—happiness, results, the love of our life, etc.—we are focusing more on what we don't have. This lack creates an "are we there yet?" mentality. Like the children in the backseat of the car on a long road trip, the anticipation of getting there is more consuming than the path and adventurous journey. Do you have the "are we there yet?" mentality? For years I struggled with being "there" instead of "here." When I was depressed in my corporate job, it was always the next promotion, the next city, the next anything but where I was that pulled me forward. I was obsessed with getting there because I was afraid of looking at "here." The here that sucked the soul out of me. The here that saturated my spirit and dimmed my light with regret and fear. The here that was depressing and a sad state of being. The here that put everyone else first and sacrificed my own desires in hopes of feeling loved and being appreciated. The here that didn't love myself. Many times when we have the "are we there yet?" mentality, we are not focusing on what we can do in the moment. We look for the magic bullet to warp speed us into our future. But because we aren't where we want to be, we resist where we are. We push against our current reality and hope it will go away. We focus our attention on others in an effort to uplift ourselves. *If everyone else is happy, I will be happy.* But then we go to sleep each night feeling empty, alone, bored, and consumed with worry. The blame can eat into our dreams and keep us playing small.

For many of us, we wake up the next day already tired from our lives, as we slip into the day excused from trying to please ourselves and failing to ask ourselves what we really want. Many of us feel detached from ourselves, so we try to please others. We fake our smiles and pretend to be happy, all while our true desires secretly mold and fester in our bodies. We suffocate our real desire by working over it, drinking over it, exercising over it, sexing, texting, crying over it. We desperately try to over control our environment and ignore our own self. In this process we develop a convoluted relationship to our dreams, we lack self-love, and we resist following our heart. For many of us, we internalize this and blame ourselves, which translates into lack of self-love.

In 2013 Dove uncovered some alarming statistics in the Real Truth About Beauty: Revisited study:

- Only 4 percent of women around the world think they're beautiful.
- 80 percent of women agree that all women have something about them that is beautiful, even if they do not see it themselves. More than 70 percent of people don't like themselves.
- Six out of ten children stop pursuing their passions because they don't feel good about themselves.

Have you ever stopped doing something you love because of the way you looked or worried about what others would say or do? This is a lack of self-love and acceptance. When we let others' perceptions and views drive our actions, we are not allowing ourselves to be fully in our own life. We hide the real us. The statistics above are directly tied to self-love. Feeling good in your skin is not about being narcissistic or selfish; it is about feeling good and loving your life fully. When you love yourself, you make healthier choices for you and your family, you focus on the big picture of your life, and you are connected to your purpose. Instead of letting life wash over you and getting knocked over by the waves, you rise up and confidently ride the waves with focus, intention, and clarity.

You, my dear friend, deserve to feel good. You deserve to live a life you love. Attaching yourself to the idea of self-love being selfish is not serving you. This belief is an excuse to avoid the sinking sensation that we don't feel like we are enough. We don't feel like we are worthy, or deserving of our desires. Instead of looking at our real pain, we are just fighting ourselves by declaring, "We don't want to be selfish."

The 4 percent of people who love themselves fully know that self-love is our birthright. We come into this world full of love. Loving yourself is letting life in. Loving yourself is not about "me over we," or sacrificing relationships to be a poster child for YOLOSU (you only live once so screw you) mentality. No, in fact self-love is about knowing with every fiber of your being that you are here for a reason, you have a light and love so powerful within you that you can't settle, you can't not do what is in your heart to express your true essence in the world. Self-love is about being connected 100 percent to love, God, the universe, spirit, whatever you believe in. Self-love is the essence of love, the energy that moves mountains inside of you. Once you dip into it, the hollowness disappears, your light ignites, and you feel more love then you ever felt possible. Self-love is not something you reach for, it is something you are. When you let yourself be who you really are, the world is in balance. Your family is in balance, your career is in balance, your health is in balance, your relationships are deep and fulfilling, you are never afraid to be alone, because you love being with yourself. Your dreams become clear and your purpose is ignited. Self-love is a gift to you.

Self-love is about the shift. The collision of preparation, persistence, and letting go of what no longer serves you, all in the name of happiness. It is the moment you step into your life and say, "I am worth it." It is the moment you wake up and the first thing you say to yourself is "I love you." Once you fully love you, you stop worrying about others' perceptions of you. My shift happened when I started to release my attachment of being accepted by others and turned inward to focus my full attention to accepting myself. When I did this, my work shifted, habits and perspectives changed, and I felt self-love. Today, I wake up fully engaged with myself, attached to my true self, and focused on bringing my light forward. I lean into love over fear and I say, "I love you" daily. When is the last time you said, "I love you" to yourself? Life is too short to be at an endless war with yourself.

The other day a friend was expressing her worries with people saying mean things about her. She said to me, "I realized something today: You don't seem to care what other people say about you because you don't need their approval." I smiled and told her that was true. "I don't need their approval; I only need to approve of myself." To be honest, it took me thirty-plus years to accept myself and learn how to love me for me. And I worked self-love like a full-time job, but in each moment that I honor and respect myself it is always worth it. People will either like me or they won't, but I can't waste time trying to convince others to love me. The only thing that matters is my love for myself.

Believe me, this was not always the case. In fact, as I sit here writing this chapter I realize how less than a year ago, as I wrote the proposal for this book, I was still struggling with accepting myself, I was still uncomfortable in my skin, and hated the way I looked. It took practicing the steps I share in this book for me to get to where I am today. My life is much different now. Today I woke up and before I even opened my eyes, I said to myself, "I love you. You are beautiful." I had a beautiful workout dancing to my favorite music, and then I went for a nature walk with my favorite buddy, my dog Tucker. This is a drastic difference from when I didn't love myself. A typical morning would feel much different. I would wake up with regret and feel hungover from all the sugar I binged on the previous evening. My stomach would be churning from digestive issues; I was bloated, headache prone, and dehydrated. I would blame myself for the things I didn't get done the day before, and be angry at myself for sleeping in. I would race to get my coffee loaded with sugar and flavored cream and frantically fall into my day with chaotic energy. It wasn't until I released my need to feel accepted by others and instead made my full focus on accepting myself that things changed. I call this mind-set "Me Matters," and this is the most joyful route to happiness.

⁀

JOY ROUTE
Me matters.

I talked briefly about the shift, but in this joy route we will dive deeper into how you can create space to allow a shift to happen for you. We cannot manufacture a "shift"; the shift comes with preparation, persistence, and letting go of what no longer serves you. Let's dive in deeper.

AWESOME ACTION 1: The Self-Love Expedition

Self-love is a wild adventure into your true self. Like any true epic adventure, it takes preparation, courage, bravado, and a dedication to seeing the journey through. Like climbing Mount Everest, or riding on camelback through the Sahara Desert, the journey is part of the reward. Being in the moment of the epic adventure is part of the big picture.

We are going to go on a self-love expedition, a courageous journey into your heart center. The love-filled joy bubble inside of you will rise to the surface, and you can feel more grace and ease with life. Self-love is about letting life in, it is allowing your choices to have meaning, and staying tall in your own power. You are worth it and you deserve to be happy.

Remember we can't manufacture self-love. It has to come from within and can only come when you are ready to fully allow yourself to be present in your life. However, this formula is what I use in my coaching sessions and in my own life. It works when you work it.

THE SELF-LOVE EXPEDITION FORMULA:

> **Experience**
> **+ Persistence**
> **+ Letting Go of What No Longer Serves You**
> **= Self-Love/the Shift**

Let's break these factors down a little more to help you fully activate this breakthrough formula.

Experience is about time and discovery. Showing up fully makes a difference. Think about when you were a student in school and you were getting ready to graduate. All of your years of preparation and experience of studying, learning, observing, trial and error were working together to help you prepare and get a job in your chosen field. You may not have known when or what kind of job you'd get, but you were hopeful and you had prepared yourself for the opportunity to be accepted into the work world. The same is true for accessing self-love. You may be called to different teachers, events, courses, meditations, or retreats, and following those nudges will be important for accessing your true self. Also know that a willingness to love yourself is all that is required for reaching self-love. As you go through life you have experiences that help you become more of who you really are. You are in the preparation phase: You are growing, learning, researching, and trusting. Be open to the unknown and enjoy the exploration along the way. Like a road trip, instead of having the "are we there yet?" focus, put yourself into the action by fully experiencing the journey. Put yourself in the driver's seat of your own self-love adventure and you will take hold of your destiny. Dive into new concepts and experiences, and enjoy the journey as you move forward.

BREAKTHROUGH QUESTIONS:

1. What are three self-sacrificing habits holding you back?
2. What do these habits cost you?
3. What are three self-love habits you can cultivate?

Persistence is about consistency. Self-love is a lot like exercising at the gym. The more you do it, the stronger you get. Persistence is action; it is about taking action and moving in the direction of what you truly desire. With daily practice, everything that once tripped you up suddenly becomes irrelevant as you step into your true essence. You let your inner light be your compass, and you allow the real you to be your source of power. Through a daily practice of constant action, you release patterns and habits that don't serve you.

Everything changes as you start to share your own frequency rather than taking on the energy of everyone around you. The shift is when you start to live from your heart, rather than let outside influences direct you.

Letting go of what no longer serves you is a daily focus of asking yourself: Does this serve me?

Life is a constant balance of holding on and letting go. Releasing habits, people, and situations that no longer serve you is an act of self-love. When we hold on to things that no longer help us grow, we become stale and bored with life. This is when the depression can sneak in and we avoid acting on our inner pull. Show up for yourself, and let go.

Pull out your joy journal and have fun diving into these breakthrough questions:

1. What are you holding on to that you are willing to let go of?
2. What habits are no longer serving you?

AWESOME ACTION 2: Me Matters

The pivotal moment in my weight loss journey was learning how to love myself. **Self-love happens when we stop trying to reach self-love and we allow ourselves to be.** Lack of self-love is connected to low self-esteem, and it is amplified when we focus on how we don't have it. I was suffocating in my own self-pity until I let the shift in. The shift was surrendering to what is and allowing myself to be me fully, in my own life. I let go of trying to feel something, trying to be someone other than myself. Instead I focused on Me Matters. Me Matters actually came to me when I received an email from a reader of my first book, *Find Your Happy.*

> *"You really know your stuff and have contributed to my healing. You've taught me "Me Matters." I love your work! Keep doing what you're doing!!"*
>
> —NICOLE

When I got this email from Nicole, I was well into my healing journey and had been lecturing and writing about my healing journey, yet I didn't have a term that summed up everything I was doing to pull myself into a happy and healthy place. Her words touched me. It *was* all about the "Me Matters"! Me Matters was a concept that resonated with me, and I began to consciously practice Me Matters. By putting my needs first and practicing what I share in this chapter, self-love became a regular routine for me. This is how I was able to create a life that was more in line with my true desires. Me Matters is about putting yourself in the driver's seat of your own life. Me Matters is about saying you are worth every drop of your desires. You are worth it. By establishing a Me Matters practice, you begin to shift your awareness to more abundant sources of love. No longer will you allow yourself to stay in situations that hurt your soul. Anything that feels uncomfortable will be removed from your life as you align with your true you-ness.

There are many ways to bring Me Matters to life. But you can put all the action in the world into your Me Matters, and if it isn't backed with solid love and intention, your Me Matters will fall apart and you will fall back into old patterns and habits.

To cultivate a true sense of self, you must get clear about who you are and what you want in life. Fuzzy goals will leave room for holes. Instead of having a life full of ditches and dead ends, create a plan of action to help you gravitate toward self-love in every situation. How do you gravitate toward self-love? You follow your heart. You go inward and begin to trust yourself. You let go of trying to please others and allow your true self to express itself fully. You no longer settle; you are happy and connected to your life. You live in the moment and you, my friend, are in love with yourself. All of your relationships are purposeful and fulfilling. You are abundant with wellness, financial stability, and inner peace.

Me Matters is about getting to the heart of what matters to you. It's joy journal time. Get ready to dive deeper with these key steps.

1. **Befriend yourself.** To fall in love with yourself, you have to become your own best friend. Just like making real friends in the world, it takes time to develop trust. You can trust yourself by going inward and forgiving yourself for all of the mistakes, blame, and self-sabotage.

2. **Write an open letter to yourself** and the parts of you that you resist. I wrote a letter to my body, and this opened up my attitude to be more accepting and loving to myself. Here are some prompts to help you get started.

- Dear me, I forgive you for . . .
- My wish for you is . . .
- I didn't mean to hurt you and be so mean; I was just trying to protect myself from . . .
- I want to be your best friend because . . .

3. Take a **thirty-day Self-Love Junket.** Go on a self-love inner journey and treat yourself kindly. For the next thirty days, make a conscious effort to put your needs first. Listen to the guidance in your heart, and take steps to follow the advice you hear. You may be guided to go exercise more, or change your diet, or sleep more. Your inner guide will lead you. Or take yourself on dates to the movies or a picnic in the park with your favorite book. The self-love junket is a journey into you. Please do this! It will change your life. When you put yourself in your life, you will start to cultivate more loving experiences and you will get everything you want. Happiness and well-being will be your natural state. These questions can help lead you in the right direction.

- What is important to me?
- What do I value most?

- List five people whom you admire. What qualities do they have that show they love themselves?
- What three things can you do today to show up for yourself more?

When we get in touch with our inner self, we naturally release things that go against our true essence: Relationships may fall away to make room for more expansive ones; we may change our eating habits; we may outgrow our careers to land our dream job, or we may become bored with where we live and move to our dream location. We will find ourselves feelings a sense of security as we leave the comforts of settling to reach for our heart's true desires. Keep honoring your own needs and trust that as you get happier, the people in your life who really matter will support you fully. Let yourself be you. Trust yourself.

You will be guided to new ways of being. Settling will no longer be an option. Me Matters is a daily dedication to you. You matter, and when you step forward confidently with your heart as your compass, anything is possible.

MOTIVATIONAL MANTRA

"I honor my needs in every moment and
I express myself openly with love."

BONUS RESOURCE

If you want to take this step deeper, download this guided audio meditation:

"Me Matters," from the *Adventures for Your Soul* meditation album. Available on iTunes, Amazon.com, or playwiththeworld.com/home/shop/

SEVEN

Just Do You

We let comparison kidnap our joy.

On our journey to happiness and in trying to achieve our goals, we often fall into comparison mode. Whether we compare ourselves to other people—how they seem happier, skinnier, smarter, more with it than us—or we compare ourselves to an older version of our own self (I was so much skinnier back then, or I used to make so much money, now I am laid off, etc.), the results are equally detrimental. Comparison robs our joy. This habit hinders our happiness more often than any other self-sabotaging technique. Comparison is sneaky, cunning, and manipulative. It will walk around with us and rule our thoughts if we are not careful. If we want to find lasting happiness, we need to look at comparison for what it really is—fear—and address the underlying issue. This is why it is essential to look at how comparison is playing a role in our lives.

It is easier to look at the outside of a situation and assume it is better than perhaps it really is. If you're single and still trying to find a partner, it may be easy to assume that someone who is married is happier than you are. It almost seems reasonable to believe that your friend who got a promotion is smarter than you. We think that because someone got the raise, or had their second child or just started dating someone, that they are richer, smarter, happier, or prettier than us. Such assumptions may be natural, but in truth, they are just ego projections that cater to our insecurities. Our ego will generate thoughts like, "You are not worthy, or pretty enough, or smart enough, or strong enough, etc." Honestly, we can go our entire life thinking that other people have it figured out, but this is always a story we create based on only a small fraction of the real picture.

I realized the effects comparison has on our emotional well-being and friendships when a dear friend texted me a while ago. He said, "I am so proud of you and all your amazing accomplishments. Your life looks amazing and you seem so happy." Funny enough, when I received that text I was actually in a moment of despair, feeling very out of alignment with myself. Of course I have the tools to pull me out, but part of being human is being in our stuff. And I was going through some emotional pain. My friend was basing his beliefs on my social media presence and how he hears from friends how well I am doing. Here is the thing, I don't post to my page or share when I am having an anxiety attack or when I feel lousy and unworthy. Believing only what we see can be a trap. A giant, thorny, painful trap!

I thought to myself when his text came through, *Sure my life may look amazing, but right now it doesn't feel that way.* This was a pivotal moment in my exploration of self, and I recognized that no matter what we do, being happy is never going to come from trying to "look" good on paper, or trying to "look" good for others. I realized that it doesn't matter what our life "looks" like, it matters how our life feels. And when we compare ourselves to people who only look happier, we're comparing ourselves to an illusion—an illusion that separates us from reaching our own desires.

Here's something to remember: Almost everything we see—especially on social media—is a carefully constructed version of reality. Judging someone based on his or her status update is keeping you from being all you can be, because you're comparing yourself to a false image and then beating yourself up when you don't stack up.

The next time you find yourself in comparison mode, remember this: We have no idea what someone else is truly going through. We have no idea what their life is like on the inside, when the door is locked, the blinds are down, and the computer is turned off. You need to remember that everybody has moments of insecurity, of depression, fear, and loneliness. Judging yourself in comparison to another person hurts you. When you put others on a pedestal, it makes you feel less than, and that may make you feel guilty, angry, depressed, and a host of other negative emotions. Certainly not the mind-set that is conducive to manifesting your dreams. Comparing ourselves to others is a common habit that hinders our happiness, but I find that comparing ourselves to older versions of ourselves is almost even more harmful. Many of us do this. We fall into the habit of thinking about our past and how we were in a particular situation. It could be about our financial status, our career status, our relationship status, or the size and shape of our body. Maybe you were happily married and now you're not. Maybe you had a successful career, but then you got laid off. Maybe you used to be a size 6 and go to the gym every day, but now you're a busy mom with more than a few pounds to lose. I admit, I have been guilty of this type of comparison too. At one time I was an endurance athlete junkie. I competed in the Hawaii Half Ironman, I ran half marathons every month, and participated in century, 100-mile, bike rides every other week. This was extremely enjoyable for me at the time, but today my workout schedule is less structured, less time-consuming, and less demanding. I no longer train for any event, and some days making it to the gym feels like torture. For many months I struggled with this personal identity crisis. I would remember my super-fit body and inner drive to compete in endurance activities. Although I still worked out consistently, my workouts became less demanding and part of me was frustrated. I would tell myself I was lazy, lacked motivation, and because of this, I was gaining weight. When I was stuck in this frame of mind, every time I saw a runner, I would mentally beat myself up: *Why aren't you running, Shannon? Get your fat butt into gear!* I was comparing myself to my past self and I didn't feel very good about myself. It wasn't until I looked deeper and started to ask why my motivation had left that things became clearer. Upon deeper reflection I saw that the endurance activities served a purpose at a very specific time in my life. I started to train for them when I was in my dark depression in Chicago working in a job I hated. These events and the training that went along with them were invaluable to helping me become happier and healthier. Training was a form of self-care—something I desperately needed at the time. The training also provided structure for my life and inspired me to be dedicated to something—tools I needed to pull myself out of a depression—and it distracted me from my emotional pain. I had replaced my misery with a healthy habit, one of training for an endurance event.

Once I became happier, I no longer craved that vigorous of an activity. It took much longer for me to be able to separate the endurance activities from my own identity. We are not what we do. Part of our despair in life comes because we refuse to detach from a version of ourselves that no longer serves us. After looking deeper I realized that trying to continue to participate with these endurance events felt out of alignment with where I was in my life. I was in the process of starting my own business, I was writing a book, and I was starting a new life. But in my mind I held on to the belief that something was wrong with me because I didn't want to train for an event. It wasn't until I gave myself permission to just be me that things radically changed. To break the habit of comparison we have to trust that everything has its own time and place, and just like seasons in nature, we have our seasons in life. The fastest way to disengage with the comparison habit is to just do you.

JOY ROUTE
Just do you.

Anytime you find yourself in comparison mode, remember it kidnaps your joy. Comparisons replace your joy with fear. But the good news is that we are naturally inclined to choose love over fear, so this habit hindering happiness can be broken, and it can be fixed for good.

The best way to combat comparison is to "just do you." This means you become comfortable with being you, and focus your attention back on super, awesome you rather than on others or some older version of yourself. When you find yourself looking at someone else and wondering why you aren't as smart, pretty, successful, etc., just STOP! Take a breath and look inward. Learn to recognize the unique, glorious person you are at this very moment, and then ask yourself what you want, and what feels good for you in the moment. Aligning with your own truth in each moment will help you become who you want to be. In essence this means you allow yourself to be your true self. Just do you.

When I did this with my own endurance activities, I realized that the new version of me does not want to get up at five o'clock every morning and run ten miles. The new version of me, the current me, wants to cuddle with my favorite dog and push snooze, or go surfing in the morning, or take a long afternoon walk along the beach. I started to just do me, which meant recognizing my needs and meeting them. I got comfortable with the new me but I could only do that by honoring who I am at each and every moment.

Whenever you feel overwhelmed by comparisons, both with other people or your own self, think of nature. As Kris Carr says, "The stars don't compare themselves to one another, and there is plenty of room for all of them in the sky." Or think of the seasons. There is a time for everything, like snow in the winter and harvest in the fall. Looking at your own life with more grace and approaching your life like seasons can help you stop comparing your current self with a past self. Trying to force yourself to be in a harvest season when your soul really craves hibernation will only cause more distress. The goal is to train yourself to tune in to your body's needs and your honest desires. What is it your soul craves? This joy route will show you how to make this an effortless part of your life.

I thought about this when I let go of trying to be someone I wasn't anymore. The endurance activities served their purpose at a very specific time in my life, but forcing myself to do them now would be going against what I need. I would not be respecting myself and I would ultimately cause more damage. When we let comparison dictate our actions, we fall into a muddy hole of self-sabotage that's very difficult to crawl out of. The best thing to do is avoid it altogether and just practice being you. Being you shouldn't be too hard; the hard part is trying to be someone we are not.

What are your current needs, and are they getting met? So many of us compare ourselves to others and we don't come back to ourselves. Well, not you, sweet thing, you are going to rise above comparison and kick it to the curb. Every time a comparison thought comes to you, you have the power to address it. This will help remove it faster.

The next time you find yourself in comparison mode you just need to remember to look inward rather than outward. Check in with your true self and really listen to its needs and desires. Honestly assess where you are at the moment. If you are operating from a place of dissatisfaction in any area of your life, you are going to see others as so much happier than you. When you compare you're just reflecting the state of your inner landscape. Recognize that and you'll be better able to stop comparison in its tracks and focus on meeting your own needs. The ones that make you happy and your soul sing.

These steps can help.

AWESOME ACTION 1: Catch Comparison

Over the next week, catch yourself when you start slipping into comparison mode. Most of us go through life not realizing we are comparing ourselves to others or holding on to an older version of ourselves. But this doesn't have to be the case for you. You can bust through this habit and reach happiness fast by catching the comparison. Literally addressing it, almost as if it were a person, you can stop it in its tracks. When you say out loud or even to yourself in your head, "I see you, comparisons. I see you making me judge myself in relation to other people. Sure they seem happier, healthier, smarter, etc., but I know that this is just one small view of their big picture." This dialogue can help you disengage with the comparisons and focus yourself on manifesting your true desires.

There are three types of comparisons. Do any of these sound familiar to you?

1. **Outward comparison** is where you compare yourself to others. "They have what I want. They seem to be happier, smarter, better, etc."
2. **Personal comparison** is where we reflect and compare ourselves to our own self—either a past version or future version of ourselves. "I'm not where I want to be; my life is off track," or "I am so lazy compared to my younger self."
3. **Situational comparison** is where you focus on how you don't have something and you cannot be happy until you have it. More money, a sweet honey, a better job, a book deal, a big contract, etc.—no matter what, you are thinking about your current situation and comparing it to a possible future that has not happened yet. "I can't be happy until . . . I get a new job, I have a new love in my life, I am skinnier."

Think about a recent situation when comparison took over and kidnapped your joy.

The type of comparison I am feeling is _____

_____

Just recognizing the type of comparison you're engaging in can help you move through it much faster. See the comparison, stop it, and shift your focus inward toward your true self. See it, stop it, shift it—stop this hindering habit before it stops you.

AWESOME ACTION 2: Go Inward

As I said, after you formally catch the comparison, you should go inward. This means taking your attention off the outside situation and focusing on your own self. Start by repeating the words, "This is only one aspect of the entire picture." Remember, we never know the entire story, so assuming what we see is the final outcome will hurt us in the long run. Go on an inward journey to your own heart. This means aligning with your own self.

Ask yourself:

What does this situation bring up for me?

How does it make me feel?

For example, I realized my lack of motivation toward hard-core endurance training was bringing up my insecurity of something being wrong with me. I would think because I am not into training right now, that I somehow failed. It brought up old insecurities of feeling like a failure and feeling unworthy. Once I saw what it was bringing up for me, I realized that the situation itself had little do with the real issue. Getting to the core of our insecurity and why we fall into comparison is the real gem of this joy route. Give yourself permission to go inward and ask yourself why the comparison is bothering you. It could lead you to your core limiting belief of feeling unworthy, unloved, or unvalued. Give yourself time on this section. It will help you in the long run.

AWESOME ACTION 3: Just Do You

"Just do you" means you get comfortable being you and letting yourself be guided by your own passion and inner desires. When you align with your own true self, the comparison is eliminated. Choose to focus on love. You are the light; you have dreams, goals, and aspirations that are part of you. And when you align with those, you realize that you are on your own path.

Part of being human is to fall into comparison mode, but staying there or letting it rule your actions will keep you from accessing lasting joy. We want happiness to be a way of life, and letting go of comparisons can get us there. One tool you can use to pull yourself out of comparisons is to align with your WHY. Ask yourself "Why am I doing what I am doing?" For example, let's say you are in yoga class, and you look over and you think the person next to you is doing a better bird of paradise pose than you. Most likely, now that you're distracted, you will fall out of the pose. Then you'll probably start beating yourself up: *How many times do I have to show up before I get this right?* The mental chatter takes over and you're in your head for the remainder of the class.

Now let's see how this tool would look in action. Instead of letting the comparison chatter run rampant, you catch it in the act, address it, and then recognize what type it is—"outward comparison." Next, turn inward and connect to why you are doing what you are doing. No, I don't mean why you are comparing yourself to someone else, but why you are doing the act of yoga. Perhaps you took up yoga to balance your mind and heart, or to make healthy decisions and take care of your body. Maybe you want to become more flexible. Whatever the reason, connect to it. This is your why. Then you can repeat the mantra, "There is a time and place for everything, and I do me." This will help you realign with your own internal compass and connect to why you are doing what you are doing. This has helped me many times pull out of comparison mode.

The best way to connect with yourself is to create a personal mission statement. I still have moments where I compare; it is part of being human. But today I practice this joy route to pull out faster. For example, when I first started my business I fell into comparison a lot; I was always looking at other speakers, writers, and bloggers and wondering how and why they had so many followers. I couldn't understand how to grow my own business as fast as they seemed to. I was looking outside of myself, comparing big-time to others. So I created a personal mission statement and aligned with my why: "I share my experiences with the masses to inspire them to fearlessly live their fullest potential by being their authentic self." When I aligned back to this statement, it brought me back to me. Those people I was looking out at had different mission statements. They might not use them or do this exercise, but my point is I aligned back to *my* why, why am I doing what I am doing. But most importantly it brought the focus back on me and allowed me to align from the inside out. When we become distracted by other people and what they have or don't have, or we get down on ourselves because we are not where we think we should be, we just need to realign with our why. It helps to have a why in multiple areas of your life.

Realign with the situation you examined in awesome actions one and two. And instead of looking outward and comparing, connect with your why. Think about a situation in your life where you often fall into comparison mode.

Align with Your "Why?"
What is my Why? Ask yourself: Why am I doing this? This being the situation (yoga, etc.) in which you often compare yourself to others. Remember, don't ask why you are comparing, but why you are doing the activity or situation.

Be kind and compassionate with yourself especially through this process. Breaking up with your inner critic and just doing you is rewarding, but it takes love and kindness. In the next chapter you'll learn how to master the art of leaning into love.

The final step to knock our comparison is to repeat the power mantra.

MOTIVATIONAL MANTRA:

"There is a time and place for everything
including me and my desires.
They matter. I matter."

EIGHT

Lean into Love

We cling to our choices thinking they are permanent.

What causes the most fear? When I ask this question in my workshops or lectures, a majority of people will home in on an answer based on their own personal experience. Inevitably it circles back to the same thing . . . uncertainty.

Uncertainty and fear of the unknown drive many people to depression, addictions, staying in situations that suck the living daylights out of them, and other self-sabotaging and abusive patterns. We cling to the familiar as a form of safety net. Change and uncertainty can feel life threatening and make us feel like a fish out of water. Branching out into the unknown is extremely unnerving, but I know from my own journey that all transformation requires us to accept uncertainty and embrace the unknown. On the other side of these changes are happiness and security. So learning to look at change as an opportunity for growth will help us in the long run.

Jim Rohn, an American entrepreneur, author, and motivational speaker, said that the choices we make in life are motivated by one of two factors: inspiration or desperation. Inspired choices are almost always motivated from the heart. When we make an inspired choice it feels expansive, exciting, and loving. Desperate choices are usually ones we feel forced into. Many times they feel heavy, uncomfortable, and overwhelming. The desperate decision is derived from a place deep in our being that screams out, "I can't take any more; get me out of this situation."

Wouldn't it be nice if we all learned to make all choices from a heart-centered, inspired place? Many of us stay in situations long past their expiration dates, or we settle into experiences that don't soothe our soul or because we are reluctant to make choices necessary to move forward because we think they are permanent. Why do we do this? It is because of uncertainty and our fear of the unknown. We fear that the choice we make could set us back, or send our life off course. When it comes to making a decision, many of us are so focused on the worst-case scenario that we are paralyzed by our choices. We are terrified of making the wrong decision. What if I told you that there is no right and wrong when it comes to making a decision? Consider that every choice we make helps us learn more about ourselves. We either learn more about what we want, or we learn more about what we don't want. We discover our values, better understand our perceptions, and ultimately, our choices help us grow into the person we long to be. Learning to look at choices as an opportunity for growth can help us make more choices from an inspired, heart-centered place.

I understand it can still be difficult to make a choice and take a step forward in life, if we don't ever know the outcome. Many of us have lived a large portion of our life making rational choices that we perceived would be the best for our well-being. We made choices based on our past failures or successes. While this method has some merit, we cannot let our past completely rule our decisions. We can't operate from a place of fear, unable to move forward because we're afraid of failing once again. When we take our fears from the past and replay them in our mind, projecting them into our future, it can make a logical choice feel overbearing. This is because we are approaching our decisions with our ego. We allow fears from the past to impact the present, and we worry that because it happened in the past it will inevitably happen again. This can prevent us from making a choice because we believe the choice we make will be a permanent situation; after all, our past has proved this to us, right? Well, hold on, my friend, not quite. The past is really just an experience we had, but it *is* in the past. When we focus our attention on the present and in the direction of what we want to achieve, the choice becomes easier to make.

Many of us fail to act or move forward because the thought of making a wrong move feels catastrophic. Our thoughts turn negative as we perceive that our next step will put us into a permanent position that we can't get out of. Think about it. Think about a situation where you accepted a new job, or got involved with a new relationship, whether romantically or a new business venture; what were your thoughts? Most people don't start things focusing on the end, because we don't want a promising situation to end. We start new relationships, new diets, new jobs, and make new friends because we want them to work out. We want them to, in essence, be permanent things, because if they work out then that means we are happy, right?

The truth: When we choose to see our choices as a permanent and a final state, it is a nasty habit that hinders our happiness. Looking at anything as permanent is a path that will get you tripped up in life. We hold on to things even when they are not working, because we are afraid of change and we don't want things to crumble into a chaotic mess. For many of us this means we stay stuck in misery. We would rather settle in a situation that does not make us happy than take a step into the unknown, just in case that next step is worse and it becomes a forever state. What if it is worse? What if we get ourselves into situations we can't get out of? The mind will run rampant along this path if you let it.

Don't let fear be an excuse not to get out of that situation because you are unsure of the next step to take. Recognize that you are in a great place from which to move forward. Allow me to go a little deeper and explain.

Several years ago, I had to break up with my own fears surrounding making a choice that seemed permanent. As I shared before, I was in a job I hated. I was a corporate-climber by day, and a depression, fear-ridden, and anxious girl by night. I was so scared to leave my big cushy job in advertising because I worried that whatever step I took would somehow lead me off course in my life. I worried that leaving advertising meant I was changing the course of my destiny, and that whatever I picked would have to be my new forever choice. Plus I was feeling guilty for "failing" at what was once my big dream. I had spent years of training and tons of money on my education just to make this goal a reality! What would I do with my life? What would other people say? What happens when everything you work toward in life is manifested, but you realize it feels nothing like what you thought it would? What if what you thought would make you happy was really just keeping you from being happy?

That is when I had to get clear about my fear and my attachment to the idea of permanence and "happily ever afters." We all have areas in our life where we do this. We stay in jobs we don't like, in relationships we don't really enjoy, in cities we hate. We believe that walking away, changing direction, or leaving situations that we wanted at one time in our life somehow is a negative reflection on us. Are we giant, goofy failures? Are we unable to make it work? We naturally conclude that we must suck at life and we are doomed for failure. We often think people will judge us and we stay stuck in situations that no longer serve us.

The real problem is we're trying to make a decision from a place of lack—lack of clarity, a lack of focus and a lack of confidence, a deadly mix of deficiencies that keep us feeling unhappy. In reality, none of your fears are grounded in truth. They are all ego projections and fear-based thoughts. When we get honest with ourselves and look a little deeper, we can transform the fear and turn it into clarity and focus. For me, I realized that I was terrified of leaving corporate because I had no idea what I was going to do for a living. I hated what I was doing, but I had worked so hard for it, and yet I had no clue what I could do instead that would bring me joy.

I was terrified, until I decided to look more deeply into it. I rolled up my sleeves and looked at the insecurity surrounding my attachment to my current lifestyle. I realized that letting go of what I had worked so hard for meant admitting that I was unhappy. It also meant admitting that I was wrong. That somewhere between the certain, self-righteous seventeen-year-old, declaring what she "wanted to do when she grew up" and giving all of her time, money, and energy to a dream, and where I then stood—depressed, overworked, underjoyed, and completely exhausted from trying to be someone I wasn't connected to—I was left feeling cold, alone, and vulnerable. That honesty is when the shift happened. I noticed that I was holding on to everything that was not working because I had convinced myself at some point in my life that this was my "forever and always" state. My original choice to be in advertising was supposed to be my career for life. After all, it was what I had worked so hard for. Why then, when I got to where I wanted to be, did it feel lifeless?

I was sick of walking around numb and isolated, so I chose to dive even deeper inward. What I found there was that my fear of letting go was really masking my fear of feeling like a failure. It seemed to me that starting over was a setback, and it meant that somehow my life had gone astray and that I was off course. What I found though, as I will show you in the joy route, is that looking inward and telling the truth about our situation and our choices are the catalyst to transformation and true soul growth. **We have to let go of who we think we should be in order to be who we really want to be.**

My focus on "trying to make it work" was masking my lack of confidence. I tried so hard to make my advertising job work, just like I did in my romantic relationships. I was pushing, holding on to, grasping with every energetic cell in my being to try to make it work. I found the alternative to holding on is the hardest part, the alternative is making a choice, and in my case, it was a choice without enough information on what would come next. That means that we have to rely on our gut instinct, and if we haven't been using our faith muscles, it can feel terrifying at first. But I found that sometimes you don't need a plan. Sometimes taking a big breath, letting go, and seeing what happens is more than enough. And that is what I did.

Once I let go of my desire to control my outcome I was able to let go of the idea that my job in advertising would be a forever state. I was so desperate that I was finally motivated to change. I was able to make a decision that wasn't based on a permanent mind-set rooted in fear and ego, but one that was based on love. I needed to honor myself, and that meant taking a step toward happiness. I stepped forward into my new life with more compassion and clarity. I left my career in advertising with a desire for change. At first I didn't know what I wanted to do, but I trusted I was getting closer. I learned that things are good for us, until they are not. By holding on to what no longer served me—a big job in advertising—I was preventing my own happiness, not accessing my full potential, and missing out on my true life's work.

We hold on to things in our life that don't work because we thought at one point that the situation that currently frustrates us was going to be our "happily ever after." In order to combat this habit hindering our happiness, we simply need to lean into love.

We lean into love by recognizing that everything is in our life for a reason, that we are in those situations to help us to grow and to learn. Understanding that our experiences are chapters in our life rather than our *happily ever after* is the secret sauce of this breakthrough. The fastest way to break up with this habit is to see that all choices are simply that, a choice. They lead us to new opportunities and to new doors that may open, but life is an ever-expansive journey where we are growing, changing, and morphing into what we want to be based on where we have come from. Give yourself permission to release what no longer serves you, and you will help yourself let go of the mind-set that it will be forever. The fastest way to do this is to lean into love.

JOY ROUTE
Lean into love.

When I was in corporate and desperate for a change, I had no idea what I wanted because that job in advertising, the one I then felt trapped in, at one point was my dream, and I didn't have a plan B. It was the shiny success at the end of the yellow brick road. I had what I wanted, and yet I did not want anything to do with it. It wasn't until I let go of the idea that my choice had to be permanent that I could allow myself to move forward. How did I walk away from a soul-sucking corporate career? I leaned into love. This means taking small steps, baby steps, one moment at a time.

Many small, subtle changes over time led to giant results in our life. Each choice I made became an exploration into my own heart. When I first left my job, I was unclear of my next step; I just knew I had to find my happy. I did that by leaning into love every day. The first rule I made for myself was to let go of thinking that whatever choice I made was a permanent thing. I would try different jobs, live in different areas, and date different people, all in the name of exploration. I would release my expectations of things "working out," because that is what had trapped me before. Instead, I became more present in each situation and saw that each person and place helped me for the time being.

What about you? In your own life, where are you holding on to expectations? Is there an area of your life you are unsatisfied with and where you want to make a change, but perhaps you worry about taking the right step forward? If this is the case for you, following this joy route and leaning into love will help you compassionately break this habit.

Leaning into love is an experience we all can access every day. We all have loving and kind inspirations that come to us. Whether it is a gentle inner voice saying, "Hey, dear, it is time to get back into the yoga studio," or "This person you've spent years with is no longer right for you," or "Maybe you should go back to school and study that new topic," or "Start saving for that trip you keep dreaming about," these are all loving thoughts. These are all examples of leaning into love. When we lean into these thoughts, paying attention to them, we can grow and move toward happiness. We will make smart choices, and we can access more joy. Making choices can feel overwhelming, especially if we don't know how the situation will ultimately play out, but when you turn inward and trust that loving, kind, compassionate voice that comes from your heart, you will find that you are never led astray.

When I first left corporate, I leaned into love like my life depended on it. I accessed my loving encouragement and followed through on everything that excited my soul. This led me to explore new opportunities, new people, and new jobs. It became the inspiration that led me to step gracefully into the next chapter of my life. Leaning into love meant I turned inward and followed a loving path. This led me to travel more, and write about my experiences, discovering my love of travel and writing. Leaning into love gave me the inspiration to start a blog called *Shannon's Sharings* to document my travel adventures. That blog morphed into playwiththeworld.com, which became an online retreat for people seeking joy. Today my blog has grown into a self-help haven for people all around the world. The website was named one of the Top 75 Personal Growth Websites and Top 100 Self-Help Blogs on the Internet. I share this not to brag or bring attention to myself, but to highlight that five years ago I created a blog from an inkling of inspiration. I leaned into love, and that's it; I didn't see the big picture at that point, I just trusted that gentle guidance that nudged me to put my experiences into a public place online. I did not set out in the beginning to make a blog that would reach millions of people, and turn into my dream career of writing books and speaking to audiences around the world, although I wanted to help people and make a difference; I just took one step at a time. I let the inspiration come to me and I acted on it. From that baby step, and then another small step, leaning into love, each step at a time, came a great reward. Something as simple as registering a domain name for a new website was the momentum that led me forward.

If I had ignored that loving voice telling me to start a blog, you wouldn't be reading this book now. That inspirational site has helped me connect with a community of like-minded people and provided a platform to share my message. Everything is connected. All of the dots in our life connect into a bigger picture, even though in the moment, where you sit, you may still not be able to see the big picture. And that is okay. Leaning into love will help you make decisions with clarity, a focus that will help connect the dots. If you are feeling stuck—and who doesn't from time to time?— because you can't see the big picture, lean into love.

Many years ago, I did not know what my career would be, but every day that I leaned into love, my path became clearer. I became unwaveringly certain about my purpose, which led me to the work I do today. Building a happy life is about daily action. This book— and this joy route in particular—is about setting a solid foundation for your future. You don't want to build a happy life on sand; it will crumble around you. This is why you must take small steps daily that will create grand results in your future. Today I trust my heart fully and lean into love with every decision I make. I trust that the ever-expansive stages of my life are always unfolding and I have learned to relax into the unknown. I am happy to guide you through this joy route so you too will have a more relaxed approach to life and so that leaning into love will be your go-to tool for making all of your decisions.

The joyful path to letting go of the past and embracing the future is accessing the love inside of your heart. When you tap into that love, the gentle pulse, the guidance that whispers to you throughout the day, you will see an amazing transformation.

AWESOME ACTION 1: Align with Inspiration

Is there a decision you are in the process of making? Do you want to change jobs, start dating again, maybe move, or go on a trip to Bali? Think about your own desires and ask if the decision is grounded in inspiration or desperation.

AWESOME ACTION 2: Lean into Love

What loving messages have you received lately regarding this decision that you can start to listen to more?

List all of the love-filled messages you received. What action step will you take to honor that guidance?

AWESOME ACTION 3: Present-Moment Meditation

Remember that there is no wrong choice when it comes to moving forward. If you feel unclear regarding what your next step should be, this mini-meditation can help. (You can also purchase and download the audio meditation to accompany this section; see details to access those at the end of this chapter.)

Return to the present moment and place your hand on your heart. Close your eyes and breathe in deeply.

BREATHE IN: Light and love

EXHALE: Uncertainty

BREATHE IN: Love and truth

EXHALE: Insecurity

Now ask your inner voice what step is best for you. Which next step will help you lean into love? The answer you receive will be loving and expansive. Trust that emotion and let it be your guide.

MOTIVATIONAL MANTRA

"I respond to every call that stimulates my soul."

BONUS RESOURCE

If you want to take this step deeper, download this guided audio meditation:

"Lean into Love," from the *Adventures for Your Soul* meditation album. Available on iTunes, Amazon.com, or playwiththeworld.com/home/shop/

NINE

Study the Blessing
in the Lesson

❧

HABIT HINDERING HAPPINESS
We cheat on our future with our past.

When was the last time you thought about your past? Probably at some point today, maybe even within the last hour. Our past experiences help make us who we are, and many of our decisions are derived from past successes and failures. When it comes time to make a choice and move forward in life, many of us stay stuck in the unchanging zone of past hang-ups. We cheat on our future with our past. This is particularly relevant in romantic relationships. When a breakup happens, it can be hard to move on and find love again, especially if we spend too much time focusing on what went wrong and how we could have changed the situation; we hang out in the regret zone.

Focusing on your past can be a problem when it comes time to make goals and move forward. Often the universe will remove situations, people, or things from our life that no longer serve us.

Breakups, divorces, layoffs, or job changes are difficult, but can be the universe's way of giving us an opportunity for bigger and better things. But they can be painful and have a residual effect that keeps us feeling stuck. We may want to move forward but our attention is in repeat mode, replaying the past. When the situation in your life feels surprising, like a divorce or layoff that comes without warning, the aftereffect can be even more grueling. We spend enormous amounts of our time focusing on what happened, where we went wrong, why did this happen, and all sorts of other unanswerable questions.

Past situations that did not work out can actually help us learn more about ourselves. What if these situations are preparing you for something more aligned with your true self? Maybe you outgrew that relationship, that job no longer served you, you were getting bored with the day-to-day deliverables. Spending time focusing on what went wrong keeps us from focusing on what could go right because of this change. When we let go of what is not working in our life, we open up to bringing in new opportunities.

We often hang out in the past for one of two reasons: We don't have resolution, or we have expectations that were not met. One of my regular coaching clients came to me a couple of years ago with deep regret and pain that was the result of a past divorce. She was sad that things did not work out the way she wanted; she had wanted to fight for their marriage, but her husband had not. The divorce felt sudden, especially because she had been prepared to fight for their love. The sudden divorce went against everything she believed in. When she made her vows she meant forever and always; "I do," was till death do them part, through thick and thin. Many years after the divorce, she was still hanging on to the pain of losing him. Other men would approach her, but she was not interested in dating other people. Her ex-husband had remarried and was expecting a baby with his new wife, and this only added to her pain. She felt left behind.

I asked her to look at her expectations of the marriage; the key takeaway was that she expected to be with him until she died. When we went deeper into the details of the relationship, she admitted that he hadn't been that great of a husband. He was very secretive and she had caught him cheating on her. She finally came to the conclusion that she was more attached to the idea of him and their relationship rather than who he really was and what kind of relationship they actually had.

Many of us do this. In romantic relationships, we often candy-coat the relationship and only see the good aspects. We see the potential and we focus on what went well. My client was idealizing her relationship as she had dreamed it would be when she first married and was afraid to look at the situation for what it really was. She had been married to a liar and a cheater, and by discussing it more deeply, she saw that she was afraid to admit the truth, because it meant she had made a poor choice in the man she chose to marry. That was the part she was afraid to admit, but the truth was also that she was taking all the blame from the failure of the marriage and putting it on herself. She also felt unlovable because her husband cheated on her. All of these feelings conspired to keep her stuck, and she avoided moving on by holding on to the good version of the relationship. The good aspects were easier to digest than facing the truth. She had expectations and they were not met. She was candy-coating her past, because it was easier to focus on what was good than face the pain of what really happened.

On the flip side, I've seen clients who only focus on the negatives in their past. This is another common defense mechanism.

We look at what went wrong and we hang out in the angry zone, which keeps us focusing on the pain. This is detrimental because this hyper-focusing leaves us with unresolved feelings. We are confused about why things ended, or why the situation played out the way it did, and we feel we don't have control in our life. Like candy-coating, this situation keeps us locked in the past and prevents us from having a fulfilling future. The best way to stop cheating on your future with your past is to study the blessing in the lesson.

~

JOY ROUTE
Study the blessing in the lesson.

The reason we feel so much pain from past experiences is that we feel like we have somehow gotten off track. Things didn't play out the way we wanted or expected. Our default mechanisms are to hang on to the good so we don't have to face a reality that may bring feelings of hurt or guilt, or to amplify the bad, keeping us trapped with unanswered questions and the blame game. Either way, we feel like we are not where we are supposed to be, and because things didn't go the way we thought, we feel off track or behind in life.

Releasing expectations is a key component of releasing the pain of the past and freeing ourselves for future opportunities. Putting expectations on our goals can hinder our happiness, and we leave little room for the universe to give us what we need. If you are frustrated with the outcome of specific situations in your life, look at your expectations of the situation.

My coaching client who had been cheating on her future

with her past—focusing on her ex-husband and where things went wrong—was able to shift her attention to the blessing in the lesson. Everything in our life is an opportunity to learn. In my first book, *Find Your Happy*, I talk a lot about life being a big classroom. Imagine if this is a school called the University of Planet Earth. We take lessons and courses in compassion, forgiveness, regret, and so much more. Situations that we go through help us learn the lessons we need to grow and become the people we need to be. *A Course in Miracles* says that relationships are indeed our greatest assignments; romantic relationships especially push all of our buttons and twist our life inside out.

Imagine that each person who comes into your life is there to help you grow and learn more about yourself. There is an opportunity to learn and study the blessing in each lesson. We have an opportunity to go into each situation where we felt "wronged" and make good with our past. We do this by forgiving our past and seeing the lessons it taught us. Everything in your past has helped you become who you are today. Looking at past situations as pathways to your current understanding of life can help ease the painful burdens of the past. You have not made any mistakes, you did not do anything wrong. From a spiritual perspective, there is no right and wrong. Everything we do in life is part of a larger picture that helps us create a deeper understanding of who we are. When relationships end, we can look to the lessons of what we learned from that experience. If you change jobs, you can think about what you learned from your past career. How did those skills help you with your new role?

Asking what you have learned from your past is a great way to remove the burdens that come with it and start focusing on actions to move forward. My coaching client started to ask herself these questions and realized that the relationship she'd had with her former husband was really not a happy one. She was hiding her true self and she didn't feel supported or loved. By letting go of the candy-coated version, she moved into anger, and then was able to release the past. She saw that she had grown stronger and learned how to put her own needs in focus so she could practice self-love and forgiveness. She later learned that her ex-husband was cheating on his new wife and was very thankful she was free of the relationship. She also was able to move on and fall in love again, only this relationship was more fulfilling and rewarding than any moment of her past relationship. In her new relationship she is very much herself and is enjoying every minute of it. The greatest gift her ex-husband gave her was self-love. She became her own best friend. She stopped cheating on her future by looking at what she had learned from her past, and within time she saw that the divorce was really a lesson and blessing in disguise.

We can train ourselves to see every situation as a blessing. When we see these blessings, we can break up with our past and start dating our future. We welcome in new experiences and embrace the present.

Let's try it out.

AWESOME ACTION 1: Resolve to Get Resolution

Let's try this out with your own life. Do you have a situation from your past that you keep thinking about? Be open to receiving guidance on how to heal the situation. Our past burdens can cause us pain, but when you are willing to receive resolution, you will be open to getting it. Here is a guided meditation that can help you get resolution. (You can also download this meditation in an audio format "Resolve to Get Resolution," from the *Adventures for Your Soul* meditation album. Available on iTunes, Amazon .com, or playwiththeworld.com/home/shop/)

Close your eyes and imagine the hurt in your past. Revisit the way it ended and imagine yourself standing in the situation with the people involved. Instead of replaying what really happened, imagine it happening as you wish it would have happened. Imagine each person said what you wish they had said, and respond to them in the way in which you felt you would have been heard. Now, go more deeply into the situation and revisit how it really happened. Feel the emotions associated with that moment and say, "I release you." Ask yourself what you can learn here. What is the lesson for you?

Write it down.

Now take a moment to go into the experience from your past and replay it in your mind as you wish it had happened. Imagine the person telling you they are sorry, or giving you the attention or love you craved in that moment.

Give yourself what you never got, if only in your mind; it will help you heal. Replay this situation in your mind, and as you experience what you wish would have happened, you energetically shift your power. By giving yourself what you never got, you have released the situation and opened yourself up for forgiveness.

Sometimes people know not what they do, and the anger you have been holding on to is in part because of the way they may have acted. When you do this exercise, it helps release the emotional angst.

AWESOME ACTION 2: Release Expectations

Releasing expectations of your past situation is the next step to breaking free of this habit hindering happiness. The best way to do that is to think about the expectations you had of the situation and then see how those expectations didn't play out versus what actually happened. This contrast is usually what causes you the most pain, and releasing those expectations happens when we look at the situations in our life as journeys rather than destinations. Many of us focus on the outcome, and when that is not met, we fall victim to the compromised outcome. Releasing the expectations and focusing our attention on the present moment can free us. Knowing that each situation in your life will unfold naturally and in its proper time can help you return to the present moment.

Think about the past situation that holds your attention and consider the expectations you had for the situation. Holding on to expectations can prevent us from seeing the truth.

1. What expectations did you have for the past situation?
2. What truth are you avoiding?

AWESOME ACTION 3: Study the Blessing in the Lesson

Go into the hurtful situation and ask what you can learn from it. What did this situation teach you?

Now send love and light to the situation and release it. This will help you become more present and welcome in your love-filled future.

MOTIVATIONAL MANTRA

"I am done grieving my past.
I let go of who I thought I should be
so I can be who I really am."

BONUS RESOURCE

If you want to take this step deeper, download this guided audio meditation:

"Resolve to Get Resolution," from the *Adventures for Your Soul* meditation album. Available on iTunes, Amazon.com, or http://www.playwiththeworld .com/home/shop/

TEN

Follow Your Joy Route

❧

HABIT HINDERING HAPPINESS
We fixate on our flaws.

The inspiration to write this book came from my old pattern of fixating on my flaws. I spent years cycling through abusive and self-sabotaging habits that kept me trapped in mental madness. The biggest source of insecurity in my life has always been my body and my weight, and this kept me from accepting myself fully. It wasn't until I dove into this joy route that things began to shift.

Over the past twenty years of my life, my weight has bounced around like a helium balloon. I'd balloon up over fifty pounds in one year, and then lose sixty pounds in four months. But no matter what my weight, I would always fixate on my flaws. I would lose weight and complain that my thighs were still too big. I'd go to the gym six times a week and beat myself up for missing the seventh day. No matter what I did, it was never enough. Even when I lost so much weight that my chest bones were poking through my skin, I still felt fat, unworthy, and ugly. When I went up to 210 pounds, I felt extreme guilt for letting myself gain so much weight, and all I could see when I looked in the mirror was seemingly permanent food belly. There was extreme inner chaos all the time, because no matter what I did or what I looked like, I was only focusing on my flaws. Even when other things in my life seemed to be going great and my dreams were coming true, inside of me it was still a battlefield of bad emotions.

When people told me I was beautiful, I never allowed myself to believe them. I recently looked at photos of myself taken over the past ten years, and I remembered how I felt at the moment each of those photos were taken. I felt so insecure and ugly; I even recall the thoughts going through my head as the person snapped the photo: *Suck it in, Shannon! Stand in the back so no one will see your body. Ugh! I hate pictures!* Interestingly, as I looked at the pictures so many years later, after I've done all this joy work, my first thought was *Was I crazy? I actually look *gasp* good in these photos*. There wasn't one picture in which I looked fat. I realized how much I must have hated myself then, and I couldn't believe how cruel I was to myself.

Those photos made me realize how damaging it is to focus on your flaws. When you focus on any part of you that you don't like, it is taking attention away from all the wonderful parts that you do like—and I promise that when you really look, there is always something good about yourself that you can be thankful for.

Focusing on our flaws is easy because society has conditioned us to always want more, to be more, and to look different in order to fit in.

I know firsthand about that type of pressure, because I spent years suffocating in depression due to the enormous pressure I felt to be and look a certain way. I was told that to be considered a success, I had to work hard and keep moving up the corporate ladder. Advertisements implied that the only path to true happiness was through a relationship. Magazines virtually shouted that if I wasn't a size 2, I was fat. And I internalized all of this, until I nearly broke.

It is time to release the pressure and relax into loving the you that is. When we focus on what isn't working and what we don't like about ourselves, it keeps us from moving forward in life. Whether you hate your body or are always down on yourself because of work demands or personal troubles, being your own worst critic is by far the biggest culprit keeping all of us from happiness.

We all do it. Fixating on our flaws is a natural consequence of being conditioned to work harder and longer, be better, be prettier, be smarter, do, do, do everything you can, be more than you are. We are trained to push harder and try to achieve more, and to chase the ever-elusive pot of gold that is always just out of our reach. Whether the pot of gold is that perfect weight, the glorious new relationship, or the promotion, we focus on trying to reach something that is not what will ultimately fulfill us. What we really need in our life are peace and joy, and that can only come when we stop focusing on what we don't like.

When was the last time you told yourself you did a good job? When was the last time you complimented yourself? Most of us are so consumed with what isn't working, what is not going well, and what we still need to do, that we miss enjoying where we are. We aren't able to focus on the good right in front of us. Fixating on our flaws keeps us from seeing the rewards of the moment.

This tendency to focus on flaws can also affect our relationships. Many people also do this in romantic relationships, focusing on their partners. In the beginning of every relationship is the honeymoon stage full of lighthearted joy and love. Over time, once the routine sets in, we begin to pick and probe at our partner. The little habits we use to gloss over become amplified with a microscope of ridicule. Relationships become fueled with fixating on flaws, and we won't let up until the other person changes their habits. Can you relate? I bet! It's all too common.

Fixating on flaws causes tremendous drama in our lives. I know you really want to be happy and feel joyful in your relationships and that you want to feel confident in your own skin. So what do we do to combat the flaw fixation? The fastest way to heal this habit hindering happiness is to follow your joy route.

◦↝◦

JOY ROUTE
Follow your joy route.

I admit I have a huge smile on my face as I write this because I am so happy for the journey you are about to embark upon. Following your joy route is the catalyst to enjoying your life fully. When we tap into our true joy, we begin to see our purpose and passion. We live with more authenticity, and the fear falls away naturally. Although this book is written in such a way that there are many joy routes that are tailored to each habit hindering our happiness, for me, it all started with this habit.

Fixating on our flaws keeps us playing small and safe. When I was stuck in my own head, feeling sorry for myself, and focusing on my body issues, I was not living with purpose or integrity. I was so down on myself, that it prevented me from actually living and enjoying my life. The shift happened when I started to back up and see the big picture. I recognized that life is very short, and that we are not here for a very long time. We have this one life that we can live fully, or we can skate around isolated, insecure, lonely, and sad. We have a choice. I decided to follow my joy.

Following your joy route means following your bliss, as Joseph

Campbell so eloquently declared. Following your joy route gets you out of your own way, it helps you access your inner heart's desires, and it connects you with your true purpose and passion. What does "follow your joy route" mean for you? Well, it means going inward and asking yourself some important questions.

AWESOME ACTION 1: Dig into Your Desires

These breakthrough questions can help you get clearer about your desires.

1. What are you really good at doing?
2. What do people always tell you that you are good at? Do you agree, or do you reject their assessment? Why?
3. Ask five of your closest friends what they love best about you and make a list of what they say.
4. Make a list of ten things you love about yourself. Bonus: List twenty things you love about yourself! (Come on—I know you can do it.)
5. What is your favorite quality about yourself? Bonus: Share your favorite quality about yourself on social media using #AdventuresforYourSoul.
6. When you were a child, what did you do in your free time for fun?
7. What does your ideal day include?

Give yourself time to really answer these heartfelt questions. They will help you understand yourself better and get clear about your true desires. Following your joy route is about accessing these desires on a regular basis. When you discover what brings you joy, you will feel more powerful in your daily activities. The world will no longer be happening to you, and you will feel in control of your world and your choices. You will have a proactive stance on your life, and it will be wonderful.

I asked myself similar questions when I first left my corporate job, and those questions became the catalyst that guided me to my happy life today. I started to write more and regularly pursue the things I enjoy. The more I filled my time with activities I loved, the less I worried about my flaws. Soon I found that the things that used to bother me fell away because I was so busy playing with the world. With that said, my weight was still a troubling issue, so I had to dig deeper.

I know you may be struggling with an area where the insecurity is particularly intense; that is why this awesome action two is so important. It is easy to say "do what you love," but if we are going out and doing what we love with negative thought patterns and self-sabotaging habits, we cannot move forward in true peace. How did I heal the negative, nasty inner turmoil for myself? I accepted it.

AWESOME ACTION 2:
Learn to Accept, Instead of Expect

Many of us have expectations of how things should be; for example, we think we should be skinnier and that our partner should appreciate us more. This constant scrutiny and focus on the flaws in our life can be dismantled when we accept things as they are rather than expecting things to be different. Accept where you are and the things you don't like about yourself by flooding them with love. Making peace with where you are is the fastest way to accepting yourself fully.

I started to retrain my brain to focus on my flaws in a new light. What once caused me intense pain was shifted to more love by focusing on the goodness that area provided in my life. I did this by accepting where I was, moment by moment; I practiced acceptance. How do you accept yourself and troubling situations fully? You become willing.

The first step is to just be willing to see things differently. Be open to seeing things in a new light, and in this willingness, miracles can rush in. I spent years rejecting myself, a thought pattern that constantly hurt me. I healed my body issues by being willing to see them in a new light, which opened my mind to new ways of living. I started by flooding myself with compassion and love. I hugged my chubby stomach and said nice things to my body. When I was nice to myself, the burdens lifted. I began to look in the mirror and stare until I saw something I could compliment. Sometimes it took a while to find something, but within time, I embraced a more compassionate attitude.

When I first started doing workshops and speaking to groups, I recall speaking at an event when I was really insecure. I was so in my head: *Are they judging me? I'm talking about happiness, but I am so fat and ugly. How can I tell others to find happiness when I'm not truly happy with myself?* I wasn't able to connect to the audience, and it was affecting my work. Today I speak from a place of heartfelt love. I accept my body and all of its gloriousness. No matter what size I am, I am light and love. I am a child of God and the universe and therefore I am love. You too are love! Inside of you are millions of love cells pumping through your veins, which are helping you move forward and focus on the work in progress. The flaws you fixate on can be removed when we flood them with love. Try it out. (You can also access this in an audio meditation; see details at the end of the chapter.)

ACCEPTANCE MEDITATION
This acceptance meditation can help.

1. Identify with a flaw you usually fixate on.
2. Go into this area of your body or life and look at it as it is.
3. See it how you normally see it, with tension and pain.

4. Now imagine this area covered in beautiful bright white, golden light. Picture glitter falling into this area. This area of your body or life is being supported with love and compassion. The glitter represents support, and the white light is the abundant energy of love. Feel this fully as you release the resistance to the situation. You are perfect just the way you are, and your body is complete. You are love and you represent light. Be light filled as you gracefully step forward with new loving energy. Hug yourself daily.

Acceptance is key!

Many people resist this idea because they think if they accept it, that means they are giving up or staying where they are, or the flaws they don't like will stay. But the opposite is really true. When you accept where you are, you stop resisting, which welcomes in new energy that can be more loving and supportive. From this new positive place you can take action.

When you accept where you are, you have a solid foundation from which to move to where you want to go.

If you have body insecurities and want to take this method deeper, you can download my Body Bliss bonus track on the meditation album *Clear Your Fear*, available on iTunes, Amazon.com, or playwiththeworld.com.

~

A MANTRA FOR THIS ACTION

"I accept all of myself,
for I am love."

Here are six powerful quotes that will help you accept where you are:

No valid plans for the future can be made by those who have no capacity for living now.

—ALAN WATTS

No matter how difficult the past, you can always begin again today.

—JACK KORNFIELD

Happiness does not depend on who you are or what you own, it requires a dedication to choosing happiness, and that lies in how you think.

—SHANNON KAISER

Accept what you can't change, change what you can't accept.

—UNKNOWN

Learn to accept instead of expect.

—SHANNON KAISER

To be beautiful means being authentic. You don't need to be accepted by others. You need to accept yourself.

—THICH NHAT HANH

AWESOME ACTION 3: Follow Your Joy Route

What brings you joy? Go inward and ask yourself what really brings you joy. When are you happiest? A quick way to stop focusing on your flaws is to follow your joy route, and that means getting in touch with your true passions and innermost desires. But know that what brings you joy may not bring joy to others.

I recently led a workshop called "Clear Your Fear." At the start of the session, a man in attendance told me he wanted to sell his house and move, but he really had no idea where he wanted to go. I introduced the concept of the joy route to the group, and his face lit up. He loved the idea, but he was having a hard time finding his true joy. He said, "I just want to sell everything, all my stuff, or donate it. I'm not sure what I want to do or where I want to go, but I feel compelled to do this. However, my children have their own ideas of what I should do and are putting pressure on me to do what *they* think is right."

A lot of us have a hard time finding our joy route because we have spent many years trying to please everyone around us. This keeps us from feeling bliss because we are focused on other people's joy routes. When we put others people's joy route ahead of our own, we will sacrifice our own happiness. This is why we feel an empty feeling inside. This is also why many of us turn to addictions or other self-sabotaging habits; we are desperately trying to find that joyful feeling we have lost.

This man's children were telling him to do something that they thought would bring *them* joy, but their joy can't be dependent on someone else's actions. When we have expectations for others to do or not do things, we place conditions on our happiness. Not only is this dangerous—if someone else doesn't meet your expectations you can't be happy—but it is also superficial happiness. Someone else cannot bring us to lasting joy.

The man in my workshop had a different idea of what he should do with his possessions. He realized that if he didn't sell his house, he would be aligning with his children's joy route and neglecting his own. Through the acceptance meditation, he released the pressure and accepted his own joy. Your only mission and job is to align with your joy route. If your joy route contradicts another person's joy route, you will find balance in aligning with your own. When other people align with their true joy as well, versus putting pressure on you to be something you are not or do something that causes you conflict, the situation will balance out. You see, true joy routes are exclusive of demands on other people. Your happiness shouldn't be dependent on anyone else. This man's children were expecting him to do something that contradicted his joy route. When he aligned with his own joy route and gave himself permission to dream, he had an even bigger breakthrough. He told me, "I sold my house, and haven't known where I am supposed to move, because maybe I am not supposed to move yet. My joy route, which just came to me in the meditation, is to take time off and travel in a motor home to all the places my wife wanted to go before she passed on." YES, YES, YES! This is the joy route. Our inner guide will tell us what the right choice is, and following those nudges and aligning with what feels the most joyful is the path to true happiness.

As he left the session, he stopped and told me, "I was pretty sure I'd come tonight and get some more tools to help me find my answer; I didn't realize I would come tonight and get my answer!" This breakthrough came to him because he gave himself permission to follow his joy route.

The key is permission and acceptance. Respect your own desires and know that they are yours. Your internal compass is important, and when you let it guide you instead of focusing on what isn't working, you will be a beacon of light for transformation as you represent your true desires and live them fully.

1. Make a list of twenty to thirty things that bring you joy.
2. Each day make sure to implement these things.

MOTIVATIONAL MANTRA

"My joy matters;
I align with it daily."

BONUS RESOURCE

If you want to take this step deeper, download this guided audio meditation:

"Acceptance Meditation," from the *Adventures for Your Soul* meditation album. Available on iTunes, Amazon.com, or playwiththeworld.com/home/shop/

ELEVEN

Nourish the Nudge

Anxiety creeps in and destroys
our inspiration.

We all have moments of inspiration throughout the day. Whether we get a nudge to go to new place at a certain time or say something to someone about a situation that has been troubling us, acting on that inspiration is the key to a happy and healthy life. But most people do not act on their inspiration because of the anxiety that bubbles up along with the preconceived ideas about how that inspiration could play into their current life.

Jack Canfield, the co-author of *Chicken Soup for the Soul*, demonstrated this idea in his seminar series, The Success Principles. Holding up a copy of his book with a one-hundred-dollar bill inside of it, he asked the audience, "Who wants this?" Most of the audience raised their hands, but only a couple of people got up out of their chairs and ran toward the stage to grab that book.

He gave it to the first woman who reached him. She is now one hundred dollars richer. Canfield asked why other people didn't stand up. Some people responded, "I didn't want to make it look like I wanted or needed it that bad," "I didn't want to feel stupid," and "I didn't really know if you wanted us to." Then Jack said, "How you act in here is how you act in life."

It is no coincidence that only 10 percent of people are in the wealthiest financial bracket. People who have a goal and work toward it are not only happier and healthier, but as Jack Canfield proved, they are usually richer.

This demonstration is a perfect example of how the majority of people respond to inspiration and the opportunity to move toward their goals. We have been conditioned to play it safe and not step outside of the box. We tell ourselves that going for what we want involves risk, and worse, we "may look stupid." Our judgments, both of ourselves and others, get in the way of our moving forward and acting on our inner desires.

Many of us have inspiration coming to us all the time, but we ignore it because we overthink the outcome of the inspiration. We rationalize about the amount of time, lack of resources or support we would get, and quickly the dream that came to us turns into a far-fetched pipe dream.

When inspiration comes to us, we must take action. Otherwise we will continue to have ideas but not have anything to show for them.

In order for us to break this habit of letting anxiety creep in to destroy our inspiration, we must first recognize that the inspiration that comes to us is coming to us for a reason. Every time we are inspired it comes to us in the form of an inner nudge. This nudge is our inner guide, our higher self, our future self, the universe guiding us. We need to learn to trust this guidance. The problem is, so many of us are so blocked with fears, excuses, and worries that we disregard the inspiration and trust in our fear instead.

We get these inklings for a reason, and it is our job to recognize the nudge and nourish it.

Over the past few years I have made it a priority to listen to all inspiration that comes to me. Sometimes we think the ideas need to be grandiose in order for them to matter, but the truth is, inspiration comes in all sizes. I remember one of the first times I recognized that even small inspiration could be mighty powerful. I had just moved back to Portland from Chicago, and I had a fight with my ex-boyfriend. I was desperately trying to remain friends with him and hopefully hold on to some semblance of what we had meant to each other, but the distance put a great strain on our relationship. As I was driving on the highway I was crying hysterically. Tears were streaming down my face and I realized I needed to pull over for my own safety. I pulled into a parking lot and in front of me was a Barnes & Noble. My inner voice told me to go into the bookstore. Without questioning this nudge, I wiped my tears and headed straight to the self-help section. It was as if I was magnetically being pulled to this area of the bookstore. The only book that caught my attention was one with a girl my age on the cover standing on a skateboard and wearing angel wings. The title in hot pink read, *Add More -ing to Your Life: A Hip Guide to Happiness.* This book by Gabrielle Bernstein literally fell off the shelf into my hands. I bought the book and inhaled every page. Little did I know that by opening that book and nourishing that nudge of inspiration my life would be changed forever. After reading the book I was so inspired by the author's words that I ordered five copies for my best friends. When the books did not come, I emailed the author and asked about the delay. Gabrielle Bernstein responded personally and said she was so sorry and asked what she could do to make it up.

My intuition, the gut feeling of inspiration, immediately said, "Ask for a coaching session." I gathered my courage and did. At the time, she was charging more than I could afford, and even though I thought it might be a far-out idea, I acted on my inspiration and I nourished the nudge and asked anyway. She said, "Yes, I will coach you." It was at that moment I realized there are no accidents.

When I spoke with her, we instantly clicked. It was as if I was catching up with a long-lost friend. After only twenty minutes into our phone conversation, she found out I was a graphic designer, and said she was in search of a good designer for her brand and a person to influence the design of her book covers. She asked me to be her new graphic designer. In turn, she said she would be my writing coach. Soon after, she started introducing me to her writer friends who happened to be internationally bestselling authors as well. As I worked directly with powerful businesswomen and *New York Times* bestselling authors, I learned about the publishing industry. This real-world experience became invaluable and helped me on my journey to become an author, coach, and speaker. It all happened because I listened and acted on my inspiration; I trusted and nourished the nudge that called me. Each author I met and worked with introduced me to more authors, and soon enough my writing and work were supported by some of the industry's most inspirational leaders.

If I hadn't followed that inspiration to go to the bookstore and I hadn't nourished the little nudge, I would not be where I am today, living my dream life. Following inspiration is about trusting that the guidance you receive is indeed coming to you for a reason. Today I trust every message that comes to me, no matter what! The more you learn to trust your inspiration, the more successful, happy, healthy, and confident you will be.

The reason many of us don't move forward with goals is that when we receive inspiration, we don't trust the feeling. Our discriminating common sense kicks in and determines the idea is not worth pursuing; ultimately these judgments rob us of joy. We let the fear of the unknown stop us from taking that first step. Perhaps you keep hearing from people that you should write a book. Maybe you have dreams of being a published author, but you have no idea how to start. The thought of beginning the daunting task of learning a new industry or spending hours laboring over a manuscript may stop you cold. Although you keep receiving guidance you choose to ignore it.

This happened to a person who reached out to me after reading my book *Find Your Happy*. This woman said she spent years being unhappy in a job and knew she needed a change, but she didn't know what she wanted to do. The only thing she really loved to do was write, but she had no idea how to make a living as a writer so she never took the inspiration seriously. After reading my first book she experienced an awakening that she had to start writing and let go of the outcome. She literally just put pen to paper and thus began her new direction in life. Now she is a regular contributor to a well-known Australian online magazine, and she has plans to write her first book. She is happier than she has ever been and listens to her gut impulses on a daily basis.

Another reason we are afraid to follow the inspiration is because we believe following it will be hard work; the thought of taking that step becomes a giant burden. But taking the first step is the only way to break this habit; therefore you must nourish the nudge. The woman who wrote to me was receiving guidance for years about being a writer but until she took her first step, nothing could happen. You see, the universe is waiting on the sidelines to support us. The universe is your biggest cheerleader. Allow it to support you fully; by taking the first step, you can cocreate and make your dreams a reality. You don't have to see the entire path to make your goal a reality; just take one step and the rest of the steps will reveal themselves to you one moment at a time.

The good news is the universe will keep showing you guidance until you act on it. This is why patterns keep showing up in our life. As Pema Chödrön says, "Nothing ever goes away until it has taught us what we need to know." The more you ignore this guidance, the harder the universe works to give you the clues. Why not work with the universe to cocreate a beautiful life? It is easier and a lot more fun. Pull out your joy journal and get ready to dive deeper.

⌒〜

JOY ROUTE

Nourish the nudge.

To break this habit, learn how to trust the inspiration that comes to you and, more importantly, learn how to trust yourself. Believe in your value and allow the guidance that comes to you to inspire authentic action.

Take the following steps to help you break this emotional habit and limiting belief.

AWESOME ACTION 1: Listen to Your Inner Voice

You are receiving messages and guidance all the time. To really tap into that internal source of abundant flow, you can listen to the inner guidance and know that it is your compass for life. By listening to this inner nudge you will be more successful, happy, abundant, and fulfilled. Our inner knowing and nudge is often our heart speaking to us; it is the dreamer that rests inside. Essentially listening and allowing these dream to be heard is the base for living an extraordinary life.

Look at your own life and see if there is an area where you are ignoring your inner voice. Take a moment to reflect on your own experience and allow your inner dreamer to play.

1. **Define three nudges that keep popping into your mind and explore where they are trying to lead you.** Is there a certain inkling that keeps coming to you that you have not acted on? Perhaps you have always wanted to write a book, travel to India, or change careers and be a wellness counselor. Of course these are just examples, but take a moment to go into your own heart and see what it is telling you.
2. **Write your reflection in your joy journal.**

AWESOME ACTION 2: Nourish Your Nudge

Now that you have identified your inspiration and joy, think about the next step. This is the part that trips most people up because the thought of making our grandiose dreams come true can be overwhelming. This is an essential step in living an extraordinary life and it is actually a much easier step than the human brain will have you believe. Just take one step, and nourish the nudge. Take one step forward and allow yourself to be present with your dream.

Pick one of your inspirations and goals, perhaps one that keeps coming to you, and write simple things you can do to move forward on that dream.

How can you nourish your nudge? Consider doing one step today that your future self will thank you for. If you want to write a book, set time aside and put pen to paper. If you are itching to travel somewhere, go online and just do some research on flights or hotels. You could even go to your favorite bookstore and visit the travel section and look at a guidebook on that destination, or create a Pinterest board and pin inspiration for your dream trip. Just nourish your nudge with compassion, gratitude, and joy.

AWESOME ACTION 3: Let Go of the Outcome

The final step to truly break this emotional habit is to let go and release all expectations of the outcome of your dreams. This means that in order to really love your life fully you release control and expectations of when and how your dream comes true. Simply trust that you are getting inspiration for a reason and nourish that inspiration by being persistent and joyful.

MOTIVATIONAL MANTRA

"My heart knows the way;
I trust it."

TWELVE

Fear Detox

∽

HABIT HINDERING HAPPINESS
We allow our fears to decide our fate.

According to researchers, the average person has 50,000 thoughts a day—more than 1.5 thoughts every second (mind-sets.com/html/mindset/thoughts.html). About 80 percent of a person's thoughts are negative, and negative thoughts are synonymous with fear-based thoughts. That means that more than 80 percent of the time most of us are putting our faith in fear and negativity rather than in love and miracles. Do yourself a favor right now. Take your arms and wrap them around yourself. Literally give yourself a hug and pat yourself on the back, because you are not average. You may see these numbers on negative thoughts, but you know that you are doing everything you can to show up daily, find your joy, and be the best self you can be. You are already light-years ahead of where you have come from, so celebrate that. The reality for so many of us is that we are not aware of the thoughts running rapidly through our minds. Like an unattended little child, our thoughts can run amok, causing chaos, confusion, and a giant mess. Many of us walk around believing these fear-based thoughts are real, but *A Course in Miracles* reminds us that "Only love is real." The goal of this chapter is to break up with these fear-based thoughts by identifying where they are crippling us. Picking up this book was a radical move forward in helping you break up with your inner critic and your fear-based thought patterns. Now we will go deeper and really look at where fear is still controlling you. Even when we show up for seminars, lectures, and meditations, and do the work necessary to create change and growth in our lives, fear will still find a way in. Fear is part of life, but just because it is present, it doesn't mean we need to give in to it. We always have a choice in life, and this chapter is all about training your brain to strengthen your supersweet trust muscles. This will help you choose love over fear in every situation.

Fear is a lot like junk food. It is convenient, easy to access, and it seems to be everywhere, but that doesn't mean we have to buy into it. There are always healthier choices, and learning how to break up with our fear is essentially like going on a junk food detox. To break up with your fear, we will be going on a wild adventure into your own belief systems and values. We will access the core of your fear and break up with it! Welcome to the fear detox! Once we pinpoint why we are choosing fear over other emotions, we can disengage and choose more loving actions and thoughts. Many of us walk around listening to the fear voice and allow it to make decisions for us. This inevitably controls our fate—and most of the time we don't even know this is happening. Nonetheless, we keep repeating the same patterns, picking the same fights, feeling guilty over the same things; this is all fear running the show.

I know from my own personal experience that fear is pretty good at running the show if we are unaware that it is in the driver's seat. When I was in my corporate job, I was extremely depressed. I was also a workaholic. I would work sixteen to eighteen hour days in hopes I would be seen by the company leaders, get a raise or promotion, and maybe then I would be happy. I lived in five different cities in a span of three years and I was getting $10,000 raises every six months. After all my hard work though, I still wasn't happy. I was exhausted, lonely, and depressed.

What I didn't know at the time was that fear was driving my actions. My corporate climb and attachment to success was really connected to my fear of failure. I was terrified of letting others down and not being the go-to person in the company. There were nights when my boss would reach out to me at two a.m. to come into the office and finish projects other people had messed up. I felt a sense of satisfaction, if only in the moment. I was the golden child, the employee the higher-ups counted on, but I was really just an achievement junkie, desperately seeking approval, and driven by my fear of failure. The reality was that my fear of failure was determining every choice I made. I overextended myself and said yes to every demand, which ultimately made me "look" good and be reliable to the senior-level management, but it didn't do much for my relationships with my coworkers. In fact, most of my coworkers weren't friendly to me at all. I would sometimes turn corners and hear them snickering about me. They sent out happy hour invites to most of the other employees except me. I would cry in the bathroom at work because I felt so misunderstood and unsupported. These feelings just drove deeper into my work, which pleased the higher-ups, but created a larger barrier between me and my peers. This vicious cycle continued for years because I was allowing my fear to control my fate. I let my fear of failure drive my actions.

Things really came to a head for me one summer. One of my coworkers was getting married and everyone in the office was invited . . . except me. I tried to ignore the slight. I was going to be working the Saturday of the wedding, anyway, so I told myself I really didn't care. I latched on to the belief that they just didn't get me, and I was misunderstood. But when two more coworkers got married that summer and I wasn't invited to either wedding, I realized that maybe the problem wasn't that they didn't get me; maybe I was doing something to alienate them. If no one at work liked me except my boss and the CEO, then perhaps I should look deeper at what I was doing to create this situation.

By asking myself some tough questions and honestly answering them, I realized that I was terrified of failing. Fear was driving my every action. Even worse, my fear was actually preventing me from getting what I really wanted, by convincing me I was getting what I needed.

What I wanted was to be accepted and appreciated for who I was. My drive to achieve kept me from getting close to other employees and possibly making friends. My fear convinced me by achieving I was getting what I needed—approval from others—but the opposite was actually true.

You see, fear does that; it is sneaky, and that is why we buy into it so often. It tries to protect us from getting hurt, but ultimately it hurts us. My constant dedication to being an overachiever and my unwavering fear of failure kept me working so hard, but it also kept me too busy to even think about what I really wanted in life. And in this way my fear was actually serving me. I was too busy to face my misgivings about the work I was doing, too busy to deal with the true source of my unhappiness. My fear-driven overachievement saved me from having to deal with the fear of admitting that what I once thought was my dream was no longer what I wanted. But fear was also keeping me from reaching my heart's true desire and living a joy-filled life.

Fear of failure is probably the most common fear holding people back. However, the truth is fear of failure has nothing to do with failing or succeeding in life; the source of fear of failure is *lack of acceptance*. People who are achievement junkies and fear failure are really craving acceptance. We want to fit in socially and we want to be liked, so we work really hard to be successful and needed. All I wanted was to fit in, and so I would work hard in order to try to get noticed. I had a deep desire for approval, but I was overworked and overstressed. My fear of failure was ultimately keeping me from what I really wanted, which was to be accepted.

How is fear hurting you? In this chapter we will explore the ten main fears that hold people back, identify the fear you may be living with, and then learn how to remove it.

There is a source for every fear. Our deepest fears almost always relate back to childhood occurrences. There is a moment for all of us where we learn to adapt by hooking into a fear, and we overcompensate to ensure we don't get hurt in that way again. For me, my fear of failure traced back to my lack of acceptance as a child. When I was in grade school, we moved a lot, and I was always the new kid. With each new school came new remarks, bullies, and people who refused to see me for who I was, making assumptions based on how I looked. I learned at a very young age that I couldn't control what other people thought of me, but I could control my own outcomes of success or failure. I dove into my studies and became a straight-A student. I would stay after school to help the teachers clean the classroom, and I felt accepted and seen by the teachers. My peers didn't like me, but I learned that if I worked hard I could be liked by adults, and at least someone would like me. If I wasn't socially accepted, I could put my attention into my achievements, and maybe then people would recognize and accept me. I had found a way to cope with not being accepted, excelling with my schoolwork and the teachers . . . which shifted my focus to the only thing I thought was worse than not being accepted—failing, and that I could control. Thus became my ingrained fear of failure.

As I grew up and entered into the corporate world, I was over-compensating with my work ethic. Although I wanted to be accepted, I would turn down social engagements to get ahead or feel approval for my achievements. This was the same pattern I'd learned at a young age; if you want to be accepted, work hard. I craved public recognition, and it was safer to work my way to acceptance than to be vulnerable, open, and to show people who I really was. After all, I had tried that when I was young and it didn't work out so well. I know that now this is just fear playing its dirty little conniving tricks, though; fear takes situations from the past and makes us think they will happen again. In reality, **what is in the past is in the past; at every moment we have a blank slate and can create new outcomes.** Most of us latch on to the fear and let it create fearful situations again and again because we keep putting our focus on the past.

Once we get clear about our fear and its source, we can see what believing in our fear is really doing to us. There is a cost and a benefit to everything or else we wouldn't gravitate toward it. This means believing in our fear and letting it control our destiny allows us to cope in one manner or another; either we feel safe, we strive for security, or we crave love and acceptance. Fear tries to give us that, but it is a backdoor approach that prevents us from receiving what we truly desire.

When we put more faith in fear than our possibilities, we are sacrificing a significant part of our true essence. And in doing so, our fear is amplified, bringing along guilt, anxiety, and unhap-piness. It's a vicious cycle. But fear not, my dear friend . . . the joy route to bust through this habit is the fear detox.

JOY ROUTE
Fear detox.

Sometimes detoxes can be uncomfortable. For example, a health detox can actually rid the body of toxins and built-up junk, but as you release these toxins and they flood your system before they are expelled, they can cause some unpleasant symptoms such as extreme mood swings, changes in body temperature, irritability, or even anxiety. We choose to go on detoxes, whether it is a juice cleanse, fasting, or eliminating alcohol or sugar from the diet, to ultimately get healthier. When we focus on the big picture of what we'll gain through the detox, we can make it through the process more easily.

Going on a fear detox can also be uncomfortable. But the good news is your fear detox should not give you physical pains or make you break out in sweats. But I will warn you that we are going to go deep and you may encounter some uncomfortable truths and experience some unpleasant feelings. To disengage with our fear, we have to dive straight into the core, and that requires courage, dedication, and a willingness to surrender to the outcome. Surrendering to the detox outcome will allow you to get to the heart of the problem. This process works when you work it, so I encourage you to be compassionate with yourself and be open to what comes up for you. I promise, in the end, this fear detox will uplift, empower, and give you the confidence to make the choice to choose love over fear every time.

When I take clients through the fear detox, they are often astonished at what we reveal. It may be uncomfortable and extremely unnerving, but as we go more deeply we always have miraculous breakthroughs. Addictions are cured, self-hate turns into unconditional love, you can forgive past lovers, family members, and yourself. Best of all, you will attract what you desire most, whether it be a more soul-filled career, a romantic relationship, or inner peace. The fear detox works!

Fear is the main barrier to keeping us from happiness. Let's get rid of it! To help you, I have created an entire meditation album, *Clear Your Fear*, to accompany this chapter. I will tell you how to access it at the end of the chapter.

First, let's look at the top ten fears that plague most people. Chances are, you will relate to a few of them.

Top Ten Fears Holding Us Back

1. Fear of failure
2. Fear of the unknown
3. Fear of not having enough
4. Fear of change
5. Fear of shame or judgment
6. Fear of intimacy, loss of self, or loss of freedom
7. Fear of being alone
8. Fear of rejection
9. Fear of losing love—dying or of losing those we care about
10. Fear of inadequacy

Let's look more closely at these fears. As we go through each fear, try to identify the ones you most closely relate to. Choose three fears to work with throughout this joy route.

1. FEAR OF FAILURE

Fear of failure is one of the most common fears. This is because we want to be accepted and to fit in. Failure is often identified as the result of incompetence or below-average performance, and this makes us feel inadequate. Many people who are afraid of failure are achievement junkies. They work really hard, including long hours, to get ahead and prove their worth through their achievements. The person who is afraid of failure prides herself on being the go-to person in social and professional situations. People who relate to this fear will be reluctant to try something new unless they are confident they will win or master the craft.

Source: Lack of Acceptance

People who are afraid of failing are actually terrified of not fitting in. At one point in their lives, they felt alienated or left out and turned to productive means of achieving and winning to prove their worth.

How It Plays Out:

The person who is afraid of failing is often overworked and very stressed, but they derive satisfaction from their heavy workload. They often say yes more than no, taking on too much, and sacrifice themselves for other demands. They could get sick a lot because of stress and a run-down immune system. They may even avoid social situations to get ahead or work longer. For the person who fears failure, no amount of work is too much; their list of to-dos is forever long and they will work on weekends, vacations, and evenings just to gain satisfaction and approval for their work outcome. They derive approval from achievements and public recognition for a job well done.

Cost:

Alienation, feeling unloved, and feeling unsupported.

FEAR FIX:

A message to those who fear failure: Recognize that in most situations, the only person judging you is you. Your expectations for yourself are extremely high, and this is preventing you from allowing close social connections to flourish. What you really want is to be accepted by others, and that starts with you accepting yourself. Work on accepting yourself by giving yourself permission to be you. Instead of doing, practice being. Forgive your past and those people who hurt you and laughed at you when you were a child; they didn't mean to hurt you. You don't have to work so hard to prove anything to anyone, because you belong in the world just as you are. Give yourself permission to play more. Your awesome opportunity is to play more this week. Turn your work into play by finding the joy in the moment.

⁓

MOTIVATIONAL MANTRA

"For today I have done enough.
I allow myself to just be."

BONUS RESOURCE

Clear Your Fear meditation album—Audio track #1, "Clear Your Fear of Failure." Available on iTunes, Amazon.com, or playwiththeworld.com/home/shop/

2. FEAR OF THE UNKNOWN

The fear of the unknown drives people to stay in situations in which they are unhappy. A person who fears the unknown will stay in a job they hate, a relationship that has expired, and in any other situation that does not serve them because the thought of moving forward into the unknown is paralyzing. For people who fear uncertainty, security and protection will always trump happiness. They would rather be protected and feel safe than move into a situation that feels unplanned or isn't fully thought out. The unknown is a lot like the monsters under the bed when you were a child; the darkness and lack of clarity feels terrifying, so hard choices will not be made and static situations will continue to be the norm of their lives.

Source: Uncertainty and Lack of Control
If we peel back the layers of the person who fears the unknown, we will see uncertainty and lack of control are at the root of this fear. The unknown represents uncertainty, and this creates a sense of insecurity, making them feel out of control and uncomfortable with the events unfolding in their lives.

How It Plays Out:
This fear prevents people from trying something different or moving into the next chapter of their life. They worry "What if I don't like it?" "What if it doesn't work out?" "What if I make a mistake?"

This fear can keep people in situations that no longer serve them and it can prevent them from growing or expanding into new opportunities in their life. They will often overcompensate to control the outcome and prevent surprises from happening.

Cost:
Life becomes stale, you feel unmotivated and guilt-ridden.

Fear Fix:

Look at your life as a big book. When you read a book, think about how you approach each chapter. You read it and look forward to the next chapter and seeing how the story unfolds. Take this approach to your own life and recognize that each ending is really a new beginning. Also recognize that all setbacks in life can become miracles in disguise. Things that feel like problems or barriers are really pathways to new ways of being. Trust that your future self is guiding you to a better situation, one that is more rewarding for you.

⌒〜

MOTIVATIONAL MANTRA

"I trust the universe has a plan greater
than mine. I welcome new opportunities
for growth and new ways of living."

BONUS RESOURCE

Clear Your Fear meditation album—Audio track #2, "Clear Your Fear of the Unknown." Available on iTunes, Amazon.com, or playwiththeworld .com/home/shop/

3. FEAR OF NOT HAVING ENOUGH

The person who fears not having enough, or not being enough, will be very focused on what they don't have rather than appreciating what they do have. No matter what they have, it is never enough. This doesn't always mean physical stuff; it can show up in habits, addictions, and in thought patterns. Someone who fears they are not enough, and who doesn't have enough, is always comparing themselves to others, always fearing that they don't have as much or are as happy as everyone else. This fear is rooted in a lack of control. These people feel powerless over their addictions and habits, and they can become hopeless.

Source: Lack of Power and Feelings of Inadequacy

People who are afraid of feeling inadequate yearn for acceptance. At one point in their lives, they were condemned or made to feel different from others. They grow up believing they are not enough and will never be equal to others.

How It Plays Out:

The person who is afraid they don't have enough or aren't enough will overcompensate, hoard, may have an addiction to overspending, or will save all their money and be afraid to spend it. They will often possess sneaky behaviors such as hiding extra food, money, or personal items, fearing they will disappear or their possessions could go away and then they won't get their fair share. They believe they don't have enough and that there is not enough to go around.

Cost:

Guilty conscience, feeling unsupported, and lacking in trust.

Fear Fix:

Recognize that there is enough to go around and that the universe is ever expansive. Being abundant and fulfilled is your natural state of being. Trust that you will always get what you need. When you can release your expectations of what you want, the universe will swoop in and give you what you need.

∽

MOTIVATIONAL MANTRA

"Abundance is my natural state of being.
There is plenty to go around."

BONUS RESOURCE

Clear Your Fear meditation album—Audio track #3, "Clear Your Fear of Not Having or Being Enough." Available on iTunes, Amazon.com, or playwiththeworld.com/home/shop/

4. FEAR OF CHANGE

Although we live in a rapidly changing world, many people fear change. As a result, they will resist it. This resistance can cause an unhealthy balance between motivation and stagnation. People who fear change will hold on to the past and be terrified of letting go. Even if the situation no longer serves them, they will focus their attention on the past instead of being in the present or planning for the future. This extreme fear of change will cause people to become stagnant and cause them to miss out on a lot of really good opportunities in life.

SOURCE: LACK OF TRUST

The person who fears change is really afraid that they won't be supported through the transition. The lack of trust in the universe's support or the natural unfolding of their life will prevent them from moving forward.

How It Plays Out:

In life, this fear will manifest itself into many forms, such as lay-offs, divorce, or even illnesses. This person will resist change, even when it is happening all around them. This makes them feel stuck, trapped, or paralyzed by their life circumstances. A layoff, divorce, or disease feels like the end of the world. They will hold on to the past because they are afraid to let go. They do not trust that life will work out. This will cause them to become stagnant and to miss out on good opportunities in life; these people will often avoid going after their dreams.

Cost:

Stagnation, lack of growth, bored with life, unforgiving.

Fear Fix:

Each new chapter of your life is helping you become more of who you really are. When you let go of who you think you are supposed to be, you can become who you want to be. Your inner self is guiding you and you will be safe through each change in your life. All change is the removal of situations, people, habits, and things that no longer serve you. Recognize that each change is happening *for* you, not to you. You can accept the new beginning and it is ultimately helping your big picture.

MOTIVATIONAL MANTRA

"I embrace the new chapters of my life.
I trust that my future self is
gracefully guiding me."

BONUS RESOURCE:

Clear Your Fear meditation album—Audio track #4, "Clear Your Fear of Change." Available on iTunes, Amazon.com, or playwiththeworld.com/home/shop/

5. FEAR OF SHAME OR JUDGMENT

People who are afraid of being judged will avoid social situations in order to protect their reputation. They will shy away from social situations to advance their career or relationships because they worry they will be judged or criticized for their choices. They carry an enormous amount of guilt and shame around, feeling as if they have done something wrong. People who suffer from this fear will often exaggerate how others will negatively perceive them, and they underestimate their own abilities and strengths.

SOURCE: LACK OF SELF-LOVE

People who fear being judged or shamed carry around an enormous emotional burden. They are overcritical of themselves and feel as if they have made horrible mistakes in life. They constantly worry about what others think about them, and overanalyze their actions. In extreme cases this can turn into paranoia; they think others are always judging them. This results in alienation, isolation, and even depression.

HOW IT PLAYS OUT:

This fear often manifests itself into addictions, self-sabotaging habits, self-inflicted emotional bullying, and staying in situations that no longer serve you. People who fear shame or being judged hide themselves, sometimes physically, and avoid social situations. They are terrified of "being found out" or recognized as a fraud. They aren't really faking anything but they feel as if the world is judging them. The reality is, the judgment disappears when they focus on loving and approving of themselves.

People who fear shame and judgment will also avoid expressing opinions, and go against their own personal desires to please others. Protecting their image is critical for their well-being, so they will go to extremes, overcompensate in social situations, and focus entirely on reputation management. They will avoid expressing themselves for fear of messing up or making a mistake.

COST:
Feel alone, alienated, disrespected, and unappreciated.

FEAR FIX:
A lot of the pain you feel is caused from past mistakes and actions that you feel were misguided. You can forgive your past and the situations that made you feel shame. Be willing to forgive all those who hurt you and look at yourself with compassion and love. You have done nothing wrong; know that everything is in divine order.

∽

MOTIVATIONAL MANTRA

"I choose to honor my unique self
with a more loving perspective."

BONUS RESOURCE:

Clear Your Fear meditation album—Audio track #5, "Clear Your Fear of Judgment or Shame." Available on iTunes, Amzon.com, or playwiththeworld .com/home/shop/

6. FEAR OF INTIMACY, LOSS OF SELF, LOSS OF FREEDOM

Fearing the loss of freedom is less common, but is very real for many people. This causes them to avoid intimate situations and worry that they will not be able to express their true selves. People who fear the loss of freedom will go to great lengths to create a lifestyle that is self-sufficient. They nurture their independence and worry that they will lose themselves in an intimate relationship; as a result they often avoid these types of relationships. This fear is often created from learned beliefs from a dysfunctional romantic relationship in their past. Perhaps their parents argued all the time and each person was not able to express their true desires, or when they did it tuned into a fight. Or even in their own romantic relationships they may have expressed a desire, such as wanting to travel more, go back to school, have kids, or move, and the dream was met with lack of enthusiasm, disdain, or maybe it was shut down. Naturally, when we express ourselves and true desires to someone we trust and love, such as a romantic partner, and they respond less than enthusiastically, we often overcompensate by shutting down emotionally or choosing not to open up out of fear of rejection, which means we can't feel free. We feel like we can't express ourselves because others hold us back or will deny us what we really want.

SOURCE: LACK OF SELF-EXPRESSION

This fear is grounded in the deep desire within people to express themselves and stay authentic to their inner selves, though it feels unsafe to do so. The fear is connected to a lack of expressing their truth and innermost desires. Fear of intimacy is also rooted in acceptance, as they fear they won't be accepted for who they are and that they will have to change themselves to fit another's view.

How It Plays Out:

The person who is afraid of intimacy and loss of freedom will spend a lot of time alone. They feel that they are better off alone because they can do what they want, when they want, without being criticized or judged. The source of this fear is a deep desire to express themselves. They often overcompensate by diving into new hobbies, dreams, or work projects in an effort to fill the void of connection. What we all want and need as humans is to be connected to others, but this fear reverses this desire by tricking you into thinking you are getting what you need—freedom in your hobbies or dreams—but you still feel the emotional disconnect that can only come with another human being.

A person with this driving fear is usually independent to the extreme; they don't need anyone and refuse to let others take care of them. They have created a lifestyle that is closed off, but they are happy with how they spend their time. They don't feel lonely, because they mask the emotion with being busy. They spend a lot of time alone, and secretly try to prove themselves to others.

Cost:

Sadness, self-blame, anger, and resentment.

Fear Fix:

It is safe to be you in front of other people. You crave independence and expression, and the relationship you seek will allow that. It will be full of respect and love. Release your need to control outcomes by relaxing into the rhythm of life. New encounters could help you accept yourself more fully. Be okay with where you are today, because showing your true colors is what the world really needs. Don't be afraid to express yourself to others.

MOTIVATIONAL MANTRA

"I am willing to accept the wholeness of myself; I express my authentic truth with love."

BONUS RESOURCE

Clear Your Fear meditation album—Audio track #6, "Clear Your Fear of Intimacy." Available on iTunes, Amazon.com, or playwiththeworld.com/home/shop/

7. FEAR OF BEING ALONE

The person who fears being alone will stay in romantic relationships past their expiration date. They will sacrifice their own needs to make those around them happy. Even when they are in a romantic relationship, they feel alone and unheard. The driving force in their decision making is avoidance of emotional pain. This means they often stay in situations that are not serving them. Being alone is the worst thing in the world, because it means they have failed and can't make relationships work. Their relationship with themselves is what suffers the most. They spend most of their time trying to please others and sacrifice their own needs. The person who fears being alone will feel insecure, depressed, and desperate to find a new relationship whenever they are not in one. They are uncomfortable with themselves and avoid spending time alone.

SOURCE: LACK OF SUPPORT, FEELING UNPROTECTED
The root cause of this fear is connected to a desire to feel needed and loved. Most often this fear is created in childhood, when a parent was absent, or a teacher, friend, or relative was distant when we needed them most.

HOW IT PLAYS OUT:
People who fear being alone will sacrifice their own needs and desires for others' happiness. They stay in bad relationships or resist living alone because they fear loneliness. But they still feel lonely, even when in a relationship, and suffer greatly because they avoid expressing their true self.

COST:
Settling, unhappiness, loneliness, and built-up resentment.

FEAR FIX:
Place your hands on your heart and feel the energy move through you. That momentum inside of you is love. Be in this moment and give yourself permission to feel the love generating from within your glorious body. You are never alone, ever; you have loving energy and support around you at all times. You can access this energy every time you put your hands to your heart. When you enjoy your own company, you are never alone. Your presence is a gift to the world; allow your true self to shine through.

MOTIVATIONAL MANTRA

"To truly receive love from others,
I must first be my own best friend."

BONUS RESOURCE

Clear Your Fear meditation album—Audio track #7, "Clear Your Fear of Being Alone." Available on iTunes, Amazon.com, or playwiththeworld.com/home/shop/

8. FEAR OF REJECTION

People who fear rejection often feel isolated and alone. They avoid entering into new relationships or trying to meet new people due to a fear of rejection. If the person is married, they will go with the flow and avoid approaching their spouse to ask for something because they are afraid they will be rejected. At work they are afraid to ask for anything, fearing their boss will decline the request. This creates an enormous amount of self-doubt and wishful thinking. They see other people getting what they want or being in happy situations and they reflect back to how lonely and unsupported they feel.

SOURCE: LACK OF ACCEPTANCE
The root cause of this fear is tied to wanting to be seen, appreciated, and recognized as you are. Often it stems from a childhood experience where you were rejected or made fun of for being different. Maybe parents, teachers, or neighbors were never supportive of your desires or achievements, or another person made you feel bad for the way you were.

How It Plays Out:
The person who fears rejection will always say yes, as they want to be the go-to person so that they feel needed and accepted. They settle in situations to avoid feeling rejected. They will avoid getting into romantic relationships or asking others out to avoid feeling hurt and rejected. They don't go after what they really want in order to manage the outcome. They don't honor their own needs because they want to ensure everyone else around them is taken care of.

Cost:
Isolation, feeling alone and unloved.

Fear Fix:
This fear is trying to protect you from feeling hurt by people who don't understand or accept you. If you want to feel accepted by others, you must first accept yourself. You have a unique perspective and gift to offer the world. Honor yourself and your unique gifts. Be willing to accept the wholeness of yourself. Align your energy with light and love. You are safe, loved, and secure. Repeat—you are safe, loved, and secure. It is okay to be you.

MOTIVATIONAL MANTRA

"I am safe, loved, and secure."

BONUS RESOURCE

Clear Your Fear meditation album—Audio track #8, "Clear Your Fear of Rejection." Available on iTunes, Amazon.com, or playwiththeworld.com/home/shop/

9. FEAR OF LOSING LOVE—DYING OR LOSING THOSE WE CARE ABOUT

The person who is afraid of dying or losing a loved one is unknowingly obsessed with the future. They spend a lot of time worrying about the inevitable outcome of death and losing what they love so deeply. This can relate to a family pet, a significant other, family member, or friend, and they may even worry about dying themselves. They cling to the past, or focus on the future, rarely feeling truly in the present. They are afraid to get hurt and therefore will often focus on the lack of things in their lives. They are unable to allow life in and they are terrified of getting hurt.

SOURCE: FEAR OF GETTING HURT OR LETTING GO OF ATTACHMENTS

The root cause of this fear is the belief that this is as good as it gets and someday (maybe soon) it will end. People who suffer from this fear don't allow themselves to be present because they fear the future and the inevitable loss they know will befall them. This keeps them from enjoying life fully and embracing what they currently have and love.

HOW IT PLAYS OUT:

This fear plays out by not being present in life and being afraid to live fully. The person who fears dying and losing loved ones may manifest their fear in many ways. This fear can result in isolation, or avoiding social situations because they risk getting hurt and losing those they open up to. People with this fear won't commit to intimate relationships because they worry about them ending. They may also be overprotective and overbearing with those they love. Many mothers act this way in relation to their children, resulting in "helicopter" parenting, suffocating the child, and hampering his or her development. This can also turn into hoarding or other physical manifestations, because the real issue is one of not being able to let go. They are afraid to lose what they have. When we open up our hearts to love, we create a space of vulnerability. Vulnerability is at the core of this fear; we feel exposed, open, and prone to hurt.

COST:

Regret, denial, a sense they are missing out, and terrified of the future and the loss that could ensue.

FEAR FIX:

This fear is trying to protect us from losing love but we must recognize that love can never be lost. It is forever with us. Return to the present and tell those you love dearly that you care for them; stay in this moment. When we open up our heart to love, we create a space of vulnerability; fill this space with light and good energy. You are dearly loved and cared for. Recognize that nothing is ever lost; it stays with you forever. Be in the moment and give thanks for the abundant love you feel. It is a good life when you can love as much as you have allowed yourself to. Recognize there is no loss, only love, because only love is real. Return to the moment and feel the love around you. Be present to the energy flowing through you; the energy of light, love, inspiration, and truth floods through you and connects you to your loved ones. Be present in this love and appreciate the moment; know that nothing loved is ever lost. The magic is in the moment, and this moment matters. Make the most of it.

MOTIVATIONAL MANTRA:

"I allow myself to fully feel this moment.
I welcome all of life in."

BONUS RESOURCE

Clear Your Fear meditation album—Audio track #9, "Clear Your Fear of Losing Love." Available on iTunes, Amazon.com, or playwiththeworld.com/home/shop/

10. FEAR OF INADEQUACY

The person who fears inadequacy never feels good enough. No matter who compliments them or how many awards they receive, they always feel unworthy and inadequate. They feel an enormous amount of self-pity and guilt. They carry around resentment toward their past and are unwilling to forgive. This is because they want to feel acceptance and feel worthy, but their fear keeps them from accessing this authentic truth.

Source: Lack of Acceptance

The root cause of this fear is the belief that no one will accept them for who they really are. People who identify with this fear are usually people pleasers and will go out of their way to help others. They will sacrifice their own needs and desires in an effort to be accepted and appreciated. People with this fear often feel underappreicated, misunderstood, and frustrated that others aren't giving them more time and attention. They will often build up resentment and anger toward those around them, because they feel as if they are giving but not receiving anything in return.

How It Plays Out:

The person who feels inadequate will never feel good enough. This is played out in their romantic relationships, professional situations, and even with personal achievements. They will pass up opportunities for a promotion or may decline an opportunity to lead a group because they worry that they're inadequate to do so. They overcompensate for their fears by trying to be a perfectionist, but remain plagued by thoughts that they just don't measure up to other people.

Cost:

Self-pity, guilt, and insecurity. This fear keeps them in a cycle of emotional self-abuse. They are often overachievers but feel they are never good enough. This causes them to work harder, often to extremes, to try to prove they are worthy.

Fear Fix:

The pressure you put on yourself is enormous. It is time to release this pressure and allow your true inner light to rise to the surface. The feelings, such as not feeling good enough, are part of a pathway to help you understand and reach true self-love. When we feel insecure and unworthy, it is a cry for love. Invite love in. Instead of running from your feelings or trying to work over them, listen to them; they are showing you a path to better understanding and love. Be present with your emotions and feel the power of your true self rising to the surface. You are good enough. For today you have done enough. All that you are is all that you can be for now; release the pressure. You fit just as you are; everything about you is a miracle. Your miraculous energy is greatly needed on this planet. You are here for a reason; allow your inner light to shine through. You belong and fit in the world wonderfully. There is no greater gift that you can offer the world than to be yourself. You are a miracle and the world needs your light, just as you are.

MOTIVATIONAL MANTRA

"I belong and fit in the world just as I am.
The world needs me to express my true self."

BONUS RESOURCE

Clear Your Fear meditation album—Audio track #10, "Clear Your Fear of Inadequacy." Available on iTunes, Amazon.com, or playwiththeworld.com/home/shop/

Understand the cost of believing in your fears is actually the thing that keeps you from what you really desire. In every situation, no matter which of the fears I've outlined that you associate with, believing in the fear and letting it control your fate keeps you from what you really want—happiness, inner peace, and fulfillment.

Now that we have identified the fears keeping you from what you want, let's dive deeper into this joy route.

Here is a chart summarizing all these fears:

FEAR DETOX			
FEAR	SOURCE	PLAYED OUT	COST
Fear of failure	Lack of acceptance	Overachiever, deep desire for approval. Overworked, stressed, often avoiding social situations to get ahead and feel approval for achievements and public recognition.	Alienated, unloved and unsupported.
Fear of the unknown	Uncertainty/ Lack of control	Often over-compensates to control outcome and prevent surprises. Prevents people from trying something different. Worries they will make the wrong move so they stay in unhealthy or unhappy situations.	Become stale, unmotivated, and guilt-ridden.

FEAR	SOURCE	PLAYED OUT	COST
Fear of not having enough	Lack of power/ Inadequate	Plays it safe. Doesn't take risks in order to control environment and outcome. Overcompensates, hoards, and addicted to spending a lot of money or saving a lot. Will have sneaky behavior as they believe not enough to go around.	Guilty conscience, feels unsupported and distrustful toward others.
Fear of change	Lack of trust	Resists change, holds on to past, afraid to let go, not trusting, can become stagnant and miss out on a lot of really good opportunities in life, avoids going after dreams.	Stagnates, lack of growth, bored with life, unforgiving.
Fear of shame/ judgment	Lack of self-love	Often avoids expressing opinions, goes against personal desires, overly protective of image, overcompensates in social situations, extreme reputation management, avoids expressing self, always feels attacked and judged.	Feels alone, alienated, not respected and unappreciated.

FEAR DETOX (cont'd)			
FEAR	SOURCE	PLAYED OUT	COST
Fear of intimacy/ loss of freedom	Lack of self-expression	Extremely independent, spends a lot of time alone, desires to prove self to others by expressing self.	Lonely, holds on to past hurts, feeling something is inherently wrong.
Fear of being alone	Lack of support/not protected	Often feels lonely in relationships and suffers greatly because they avoid expressing their true self. Sometimes they stay in bad relationships or resist living alone due to their fear of lonliness.	Settling, unhappy, lonely, built-up resentment.
Fear of rejection	Lack of acceptance	Says yes all the time. Settles in situations to avoid rejection; doesn't go after what they really want so they can manage outcomes. Doesn't say no or honor their own needs; afraid of asking for what they want. Life situations stay the same and they are miserable.	Feels isolated, alone, and unloved.
Fear of dying/ losing those we care about	Not being present / Afraid to live	Clings to the past; often doesn't express true feelings, afraid to get hurt, focused on areas of	Regret, denial, self-hate.

FEAR	SOURCE	PLAYED OUT	COST
		deficiency and worries about the future, not the present. Not able to fully allow life in.	
Fear of inadequacy	Lack of acceptance	Perfectionist, often avoids being vulnerable and expressing real self. Plagued by thoughts that they just don't measure up to other people. Always comparing. Extreme self-sabotage.	Self-pitying, guilt-ridden, insecure.

FEAR FIX

FEAR	MOTIVATIONAL MANTRA
Fear of failure	For today I have done enough. I allow myself to just be.
Fear of the unknown	I trust the universe has a plan greater than mine. I welcome new opportunities for growth.
Fear of not having enough	Abundance is my natural state; there is plenty to go around.
Fear of change	I embrace the new chapter of my life. I trust that my future self is gracefully guiding me.
Fear of shame / judgment	I choose to honor my unique self with a more loving perspective.

FEAR FIX (cont'd)	
FEAR	MOTIVATIONAL MANTRA
Fear of intimacy/ losing self/ loss of freedom	I am willing to accept the wholeness of myself. I express my authentic truth with love.
Fear of being alone	If I want others to love me for me, I must love myself first. I am my own best friend.
Fear of rejection	It is safe to be me.
Fear of dying / losing those we care about	I allow myself to fully feel this moment. I welcome life in.
Fear of inadequacy	I belong and I fit in this world just as I am.

AWESOME ACTION 1: Fear Detox

Identify the three fears you relate to most and how each has played out in your life.

1. My top 3 fears are:

    *   _____

    *   _____

    *   _____

2. How have these fears played out in your life?

FEAR	PLAYED OUT
Example: Fear of Failure	I overachieve at work, often alienate potential new relationships, etc.

AWESOME ACTION 2: Road to Recovery

Identify the cost of each of your fears and then the benefit. How has believing in that fear helped you cope with painful situations?

FEAR	COST OF BELIEVING THIS FEAR	BENEFIT (HOW HAS IT HELPED ME COPE?)
Fear of failure	People talk behind my back, I feel alone.	I can control the amount of pain I endure by working harder to please my boss. I get approval from management.

AWESOME ACTION 3: Break up with Your Fear

In order to break up with our fear, we have to go back to the source, the reason the fear started in the first place. This requires a deep dive into your childhood. Most of our fears start when we are little and become a coping mechanism to help us relate to and feel protected from the world.

From the list above, use your top three fears and get to the sources that caused them.

FEAR	SOURCE	SITUATION OF SOURCE
Fear of failure	Lack of acceptance	What happened in your childhood where you didn't feel acceptance?
Fear of the unknown	Uncertainty/ lack of control	What happened in your childhood where you felt out of control and uncertain of the outcome?
Fear of not having enough	Lack of power/ inadequacy	What happened in your childhood where you felt a lack of power and inadequate?
Fear of change	Lack of trust	What happened in your childhood where a change created an unwanted outcome?

FEAR	SOURCE	SITUATION OF SOURCE
Fear of shame OR judgment	Lack of self-love	What happened in your childhood where you felt criticism for expressing your true self?
Fear of intimacy OR loss of freedom	Lack of self-expression	What happened in your life where you felt unsupported or accepted for being who you are?
Fear of being alone	Lack of support/not protected	What happened in your life where you felt exposed and vulnerable?
Fear of losing love—dying or losing those you care about	Not being present/afraid to live	What happened in your life where you regretted not saying or doing something, and then it was too late?
Fear of inadequacy	Lack of acceptance	What happened in your life where you felt alienated or left out?

After you identify the source of each fear, the best way to break up with it is to forgive! Amen, buddy, you read that correctly! Forgiveness is the path to freedom in this joy route. By identifying the situation that occurred in your past, you can re-create the outcome and eliminate the fear. Forgiveness is about setting you free of the emotional burdens and releasing the energetic hold. When you go back to the source and forgive those that hurt you, alienated you, abandoned you in a time of need, or mistreated you in any manner, you allow yourself to release the coping mechanism of your fear. Remember, it works when you work it, so try it out. Seriously, visualize the situation that caused you pain and surround it with white light. Give an emotional hug to each person who hurt you. Allow the situation to play out in your mind in a more loving manner. Give yourself the attention, the love, the support that you never received from those who hurt you.

The final joyful way to break up with your fear is to repeat the motivational mantra that is tied to your fear. Repeat the mantras daily, and at every moment the fear-based voice creeps in. By practicing these more loving thoughts, you will disengage with your fear and step into a more miraculous life.

BONUS RESOURCE

If you want to take this step deeper, download this guided audio meditation album:

Clear Your Fear meditation album. Available on iTunes, Amazon.com, or playwiththeworld.com/home/shop/

THIRTEEN

Go on an Abundance Adventure

HABIT HINDERING HAPPINESS
We "should" all over ourselves.

When is the last time you said, "I should do something"? Most of us fall into "should" all the time, and we end up "should-ing" all over ourselves. "I should work out," "I should call him back," "I should spend more time with my family." "I should . . ." We put a lot of pressure on ourselves to do things that may not align with what we really want to do. "Should-ing" all over ourselves happens in our work life, our relationships, our health and lifestyle; it happens because we spend more time allowing society and others to tell us what to do instead of honoring our own internal compass.

"Should-ing" all over ourselves is a constant push/pull as we fight our inner desires to meet the demands of the world. When you say you should do something, it creates a pull effect on your energy; there is a demand that can put unnecessary pressure on your life. For the next seven days, notice how often you say "should"; replace this word with "could" and watch what happens.

Using the word "could" in place of "should" will open new opportunities.

Instead of saying, "I should work out," tell yourself, "I could work out." Suddenly you will feel as if you are giving yourself a choice. The natural tendency when giving a choice is to follow through with action. "Could" is a magic little word that can remove emotional blocks and help you feel more free.

Although humans crave choice, we don't like indecision. If we have too many choices, we can become paralyzed and fail to move forward. A fantastic demonstration of too many choices that cause indecision is the toothpaste aisle. Have you ever tried to buy a new type of toothpaste? Not only are there different brands but there are also different flavors, and different types within those types, and then more subtypes beyond those. Do you want a gel or paste, anti-decay, desensitizing, anti-plaque, whitening, herbal, all natural, gum disease protection, cavity protection, tooth powder . . . ? Oh, my head is spinning! According to a piece in the *Wall Street Journal,* in 2008, over 400 toothpaste brands were sold and in 2007 alone, over 100 new toothpaste brands were created. That is a new brand created every three days.

With all of the choices in our world, it always comes back to picking the toothpaste that you like and one you know you will use. This is the same way to approach choices in your life. When you are pressed to make a decision, replace "I should . . ." with "I could . . ." and follow your way to happiness with the choice that feels most joyful.

When it comes to toothpaste, ultimately, I just want my teeth clean. With so many choices, I often dread going to the aisle because I am overwhelmed by possibilities and I have no idea which one will be the best. That was the case until I changed my "should" into "could." Instead of saying, "I should buy toothpaste," I said, "I could find a new toothpaste," and this created a mini-adventure as I went into it with an open mind. Replacing the word "should" with "could" works for little choices like toothpaste, but it also works for big life choices; things like breaking up with a partner, changing jobs, or moving to a new city. "Could" yourself to new possibilities, and it will help you feel more empowered.

One of my life-coaching clients came to me full of regret and fear. In our first session, she expressed how much pressure she was under to care for her mom after her father had died. She quit school to move home to "do the right thing" and be there for her mother. Three years later, she was unhappy, regretful, and hanging on to the "should." She felt she should be a "good girl" and put her dreams aside to make sure everyone else around her was happy and cared for. What she did was "should" her way into a depression. When we met she was bored with life, angry at the world, and unable to find her inner dreamer. She had no idea what she wanted, she just kept falling into the demands of being an adult and meeting the extremely grueling expectations of the "should." I encouraged her to catch herself when she said "I should" and replace it with "I could." This small step reaped tremendous results. Within a couple of weeks, I saw her inner light shine through. She was smiling, her eyes were full of life again, and she was dreaming much bigger. Her "could" allowed her to see that she was not trapped, and that life was not happening to her. She had control and could steer herself in a direction that felt more joyful. Within a few months, she had the clarity to approach her dream career of being a travel photographer and took herself on a trip to the Dominican Republic. She explored new opportunities in life and opened herself up to living it more fully. She sent me photos she took of herself paddleboarding into the sunset with the caption, "Healing the soul, I found my happy, thank you."

The process of replacing "should" with "could" can help you align with your authentic truth. In many situations you will find that what you think you should do is not the best thing, while other times it might be. When you feel like you are giving yourself a choice, it brings clarity and freedom. The best way to allow yourself to embrace new opportunities is to go on an abundance adventure.

～

JOY ROUTE
Go on an abundance adventure.

Replacing your "should" with "could" is a great first step to opening yourself up to new possibilities. If you are in a position where you feel stuck and uncomfortable with your outcomes, ask yourself if you have been saying "should." The world "should" can hinder our happiness even when we say things like "I should be happier," or "I shouldn't be sad." Being present with your feelings is an important step in self–love. Respecting yourself means experiencing your feelings fully. When we say we should or should not feel a specific way, we may be going against our real emotional guidance system, which can cause more pain and inner turmoil.

On my own journey to wellness and happiness, the "should" was my default word. I carried it around, slipping it into every thought and situation. "I should work out," "I should be happier," "I shouldn't be sad," "I should be more successful," etc. The "should" ate me alive and put an enormous amount of pressure on me. This led me to overeat and binge at night, which led me to pile on more guilt, and I would feel even worse.

After crying myself to sleep one too many times, I asked myself, "Why can I teach people how to be happy, but not feel really happy in my own right?" The answer came like a booming inner roar; it was my inner voice, but it sounded like what I imagine God would sound like—authoritative, demanding, and matter-of-fact. It said, "You aren't allowing yourself to be happy!" All of a sudden a huge weight lifted from my shoulders, and I saw that the only thing keeping me from being happy was my own unwillingness to feel it fully.

My pattern of not allowing happiness in my life was a residual habit left over from my days of depression. When I was depressed in my corporate job, I said "should" all the time. "I have everything I want. I should be happy. What's wrong with me?" I suspect that I am not alone; many of us try to get happy, but spend so much time "trying" that we never quite get there. The truth is that if we stopped trying to be happy, we could access the happiness we already have within. We could see that we are naturally happy, and that happiness is part of experiencing and living life fully. When we let go of "should," we can dive into our real happiness, which your authentic self will always choose.

It is easier to replace our "should" when we go on an abundance adventure. An abundance adventure is the release of trying to get happy, and instead focusing on the happiness within. I found that it is the chase for happiness that keeps us in this thirsty quest— wanting, pining for, and craving happiness. We suffocate our innate happiness and create our own depression. For many of us, chasing happiness is our drug of choice. It is easier to admit we are sad, miserable, or reaching for something we don't yet have, than to admit we have arrived. Admitting we are happy means we've succeeded. What's so bad about that, you ask? When we allow ourselves to be happy, you may wonder, *Now what? Is life over? Does it go downhill from there?* Once we reach what we work so hard to get, then what? And for many, that's a scary question.

I realized my attachment to feeling sad, and not fully allowing myself to own my happiness was no longer serving me. I also found that it became easier to let go when I went on an abundance adventure. I asked myself the following questions.

AWESOME ACTION 1: Execute Your Excuses

Many of us hang on to excuses and reasons that prevent us from reaching what we really want. Instead of putting enormous pressure on yourself to be everything to everyone, ask these strategic questions to help you release the excuses preventing you from joy.

- What reasons are you holding on to that are keeping you from your goal?
- What is in your life that is no longer serving you?
- What thought patterns and habits do you keep falling into?
- How have those patterns prevented you from being happy?
- Are you giving yourself credit for all the awesomeness you are doing?

Be proud of how far you've come, because you are doing amazing work.

AWESOME ACTION 2:
Go on an Abundance Adventure

After you analyze your excuses and see them as fear-based thoughts, you can reach for new, feel-good actions that will reap real results. The abundance adventure is all about you and your heart's desires. You can replace your "should" with "could" when you are clear about the options that exist.

These questions can help you dive into your own abundance adventure. As you go through these questions, it is best to pick one situation that you feel trapped or stuck in as an example to work through.

1. Where have you been saying, "I should" in this situation?
2. How have the "shoulds" played out and hindered you from being happy?
3. Replace your "should" with "could" and list alternatives to the scenario.

For example:

SITUATION:
I feel stuck in life because I can't seem to lose weight. I weigh more than I ever have, and my clothes don't fit. I feel hopeless, ugly, and fat.

1. The "should":
   - I have been saying I should eat less, and go to the gym, where I should work out longer. I should stop eating sugar and french fries.
2. The result:
   - My "should" has played out in late-night binges. I feel guilty for overeating, and then I say I should wake up in the morning and exercise, but I am so tired I push snooze and then I am late to work. I feel ashamed because I can't seem to find the motivation to work out, and my "should" keeps me feeling unloved and unsupported.
3. Replace "should" with "could":
   - Instead of saying I should work out at the gym, I say I could go for a longer walk with my dog and/or children. Instead of saying I should stop eating sugar, you say I could focus on drinking a glass of sparkling water during a food craving. Instead of saying I should stop eating ice cream, I could eat Greek frozen yogurt, still creamy but healthier for me.

The abundance adventure is about replacing your doubts with confidence and clarity. As you explore new options, you will reach your goals with a more compassionate approach. Stop putting so much pressure on yourself to do things that don't feel aligned with your inner light. The abundance adventure gives you permission to be you. It gives you choices. And when you have choices that are inspired by loving intentions you will make smarter, healthier decisions—ones that align with your true self.

⁓

MOTIVATIONAL MANTRA

"I make choices from a place of inspiration.
I do what feels right for me in every moment."

FOURTEEN

Rock the Reflection

HABIT HINDERING HAPPINESS
We take it personally.

One of my goals when I left the corporate world was to create a business that was location independent. I wanted to be able to work from anywhere in the world, traveling, writing, and speaking in places all around the globe. As this goal manifested, I started to see a shift in some of my friends. Some of them were not as supportive as I had hoped, and some of them were downright hostile. Even now I see people in my life shift when I share my dreams with them.

One of my visions was to write this book in one of my favorite places in the world, Hawaii. I told a friend about my plans and I naturally assumed that she would be happy for me; after all, I am following my heart and living my dreams. When my friend responded with, "You are so selfish and only think about yourself! You'll be back in a month because it is so expensive there!" I was shocked. My friend of the past fourteen years told me I was selfish for following my heart? The entire story is that she had called to invite me to her birthday party in Las Vegas. I said, "I probably won't be able to go because I will have just arrived in Hawaii, and to fly back at that time would be out of my budget." I told her I loved her, and that it had nothing to do with her, but that I couldn't commit 100 percent; that is why she called me selfish. You see she was taking it personally. She was thinking that because I couldn't make it to her birthday party in Vegas that I was saying I didn't think she was important or worth showing up for. Of course, I didn't mean this at all; she was putting words into my mouth, attributing a hidden meaning to what I said. When I said I couldn't make it, it had nothing to do with her at all; it was just bad timing for a trip.

Many of us do this; we put meaning into what other people say and do. We take things personally. We put expectations on friends to be a certain way and do things that we think they should do, because we would if we were in that situation. Granted, my friend is the type of person who would drop everything at any time to be there for her friends, even if it put her into debt. Since I have shifted gears to focus on my own well-being and grounding myself in my career and getting my health in order, my priorities are not aligned with hers. She just wanted me to show up for her in the way she would have shown up for me. However, I needed to remain true to my inner guidance.

When we put expectations on others, we're setting ourselves up for disappointment and diminishing our own value. When we demand that others show up for us as we would for them, and they don't do it, we fall victim to the energy of unworthiness. We attribute emotions to their actions, assuming that they don't care, that we don't matter to them, that they think we are unimportant. We take it personally. Have you ever said or had someone say to you, "If you really loved me you would, x, y, or z"? The reality is we are putting conditions on our love and expecting people to do things based on what we think is loving, but each individual speaks a different love language.

What I wanted was support. What I got was disdain and rejection. I admit, I did take it personally at first. I thought, *How come my friend of fourteen years isn't being supportive? I am following my heart, she doesn't care about me, and she only cares about herself!* Did you catch what just happened there? I was actually holding energetic emotions that were completely aligned with hers. She called me selfish and said I only cared about myself, and when I was in the energy of taking it personally, I was reflecting that too. I was carrying around the mentality that my friend was being selfish for not being happy for me that I was moving to my dream location. I had to check myself because I was on a one-way fast track to "Woe-is-me-ville." I had to stop and release my judgment of her because I was hurt, and I was expecting her to be someone she isn't. She in turn was expecting me to be someone I am not. We were both putting conditions on the relationship, which caused the drama. We were both expecting each other (even if we didn't outwardly say it) to do what we wanted for ourselves: She wanted me to come to her party, and I wanted her to be happy about my move to Hawaii. Neither of us got what we wanted because we were focusing on how much the other person hurt us.

Maybe you can relate. Have you ever told someone about your dreams and they reacted less than supportively? This happens a lot when we start making goals and start to achieve them. Maybe you have been working really hard and trying to get noticed by a significant other or your boss and they don't respond in the way you would like, and you are stuck right now, taking it personally. It is hard not to take things personally, because we are human beings with real emotions. But we'd be much better off if we were able to recognize that most of the time, someone else's reaction has really nothing to do with us. Their reactions are all about them.

Whatever your goal—perhaps you have decided to travel to Bali for a few months, quit your corporate job (go, you, go!), or you are finally ready to write that novel—dreams take courage. Dreaming can be risky, and when we act on our dreams, the risk is amplified in others. Dreamers set the stage for what is possible, they paint a picture of an ideal life, and you will find that for some people in your life this creates fear and frustration as they battle with their own lost hopes and desires.

Many of us don't give ourselves permission to dream. It is too risky and we say things like, "I might fail!" This keeps us locked into the fear danger zone. If you are dreaming, you are a visionary, someone stepping into the brave new world of "I MATTER and my dreams are worth it." Give yourself credit! What you are doing is amazing! When you start following through on your dream it can bring up reactions from others. We can't expect everyone to get on board with our desires. That's not what life is about. If everyone got along perfectly and had the exact same dream, we would be bored out of our minds. Embrace the contrasts in life. We are here to enjoy the diversity and appreciate the contrasts. Taking it personally contradicts the reason we are here. We want to enjoy life and live it fully, but if we are spending our time walking on eggshells, or bending over backward for others, we are not able to move gracefully into our own desires.

Your job and mission as a dreamer is not to be derailed by unsupportive people; most essentially, you must not take things personally. As you begin to practice the principles shared in this book, and you start to show up for yourself more, you may see a shift in those around you. I talk a lot about this in my first book,

Find Your Happy, where I call friends who are unsupportive social vampires. They are people who only want to talk about themselves and the gossip in their life. The moment I started to live my dreams, many of them reacted negatively. There was even an ex-boyfriend and a formerly close friend who started an "I Hate Shannon Club." I could easily have been affected by that, but I had to learn how to align myself with the light. When we don't take things personally, we are aligned with what really matters—love and compassion. We can't fight hate with hate, so if there is a person who is reacting negatively or unsupportively to you, you don't have to take it personally, it has nothing to do with you.

A while ago I wrote an article that was picked up by the Australian online newspaper *News.com.au* called "The 25 Things Happy People Do Differently"; this article took off like wildfire. I remember coming out of yoga one night and seeing over 700 new Facebook Likes on my author page, Shannon Kaiser Writes. I had over 1,000 new subscribers to my newsletter, 140 new emails from people saying thank you and asking to work with me. This one article led to three international radio interviews and two TV interviews. It was an awesome reaction, but with the enormous success of this article came a lot of backlash. There were Twitter haters, Facebook sabotages, and I found an entire website dedicated to bashing this article and me. The author took each of the twenty-five points and contradicted them to the best of his ability. Now this is something I could have taken personally. I could have focused on the haters and negative backlash, but I chose to take the high road. I aligned myself with love and connected to my truth. I knew that I had integrity (always) in writing the article and was thankful for the people my message touched. I only held space for the good; I was able to turn my attention away from the darkness because I was connected to the light. The site was removed and the negative haters disappeared and moved on to another person to harass. I didn't take it personally and the situation went away.

If someone says something to you, and you feel unsupported or attacked, the first step is to recognize that it has nothing to do with you. What people say and do is about them, not you. When I said no to my friend's birthday party in Las Vegas, it was about me getting settled in Hawaii and saving my money; it wasn't about her. My online bullies were about them, not me. When I refused to give attention to the drama, it went away completely. What drama in your life can you refuse to give attention to?

You might be reading this and thinking about people in your life who are taking things personally, but chances are you might also find an area of your life where you are taking things personally. We can't escape this habit; it is part of being human. But we can condition our rock star inner faith muscles to lift up and block out any troubling situation, and the best way to do this is to rock the reflection.

JOY ROUTE
Rock the reflection.

Whenever you feel like a loved one is being unsupportive of you, either you are taking things personally, or others are taking it personally—probably both. The fix is to rock the reflection. This means you literally hold up an energetic mirror and see what is reflected in your situation. Ask yourself, "What can I learn here?"

I learned:

1. What people say is a reflection of their thoughts and fears not yours.

2. Following your heart and making your dreams come true can make some people extremely uncomfortable.

I also asked myself, "What bothers me most about this situation?" I realized that I was upset because she wasn't supporting my life goal being actualized. Moving to Hawaii was a really big dream of mine, and she was not happy for me. By holding up the energetic mirror, I recognized that I wasn't supporting her either. She wanted her good friend to come to Vegas for her birthday—this was *her* big dream! This was her Hawaii. I didn't see the importance to her of her party in Vegas, and she didn't see the importance to me of my move to Hawaii. We were actually just reflecting each other. I was thinking she was selfish and she was telling me I was selfish. Once I rocked the reflection, it healed the situation completely. Rock the reflection means you show up fully and be proactive about your role in the situation.

It has been said that what we dislike in others is a reflection of an area of our life that we are not willing to look at; this is the mirror technique or, as I call it, rock the reflection. This joy route will help you go a little deeper.

AWESOME ACTION 1: Discover Your Deep Desires

The more confident we are in our own dreams, the less we waver when others are unsupportive. We take it extremely personally when they do or say things in conflict with our dreams, and we start to waver under their criticism.

The first part of rock the reflection is to get in touch with your own desires. When you start to dream bigger you make way for your own expansiveness. What others say and do will no longer affect you. You will be so connected to your truth that their opinions won't derail you one bit.

Be confident in your own heart's desires. Your dreams matter and they are part of you for a reason. The more confident you are in your dreams, the less you will need others' approval. If you are going to other people hoping they will support and approve of your goal, move on! The truth is, not everyone will support you. Guess what though? That is perfectly okay. Just as you might not understand why someone wants to achieve his or her dream, others might not understand your dreams. It doesn't mean anyone's dreams are "wrong." Each person's dream is unique to them, and the best thing you can do as a supportive friend and fellow dreamer is to be happy for other dreamers; support them in what makes them happy and do things in your own life that make you happy. Stop trying to please everyone by sacrificing yourself. As a dreamer, your job is not to get everyone on board with your plan, but to actualize your plan. Focus on actionable steps that will make your goals a reality.

1. What is your biggest desire?
2. What three steps can you put into motion to actualize your dreams this week?

AWESOME ACTION 2: Focus on the Results

Are you in reasons or results mode? Your focus will predict your success. Instead of listening to my friend's reasons why moving to Hawaii was a bad idea, I focused my attention on the results I wanted to achieve: to wake up and surf in the warm ocean; to be sun kissed and return to my fit, lean self; to be inspired by nature and the Aloha life. These things jazz me up; what jazzes you up? Find the results you want and your reasons will fall away fast. Instead of focusing on the reasons your goal is not coming true, focus on the results you want to feel.

The more I step into my ideal life, the more I learn about those around me. When you share your dream with others and they don't support you, it has nothing to do with you. People's reactions most often reflect their own insecurities and fears. Be okay with not having everyone's approval; the only thing that matters is that you approve of your own actions.

If you are dreaming and looking for support for your dreams, turn inward. Your heart will be the best cheerleader to help you get to where you really want to be. When you start leading your life with your dreams in full focus, you will see those people in your life that really matter rise with you and fully support you.

Remember, the more connected you are to your dreams, the less other people's opinions will matter. You won't fall into taking it personally when you have your own approval within.

What results do you want to feel from reaching your goals?

AWESOME ACTION 3: Rock the Reflection

The final fun step is to literally rock the reflection by going deep into the situation that is causing you frustration. Do you have a friend who is unsupportive or a significant other or boss who is not showing up for you the way you want them to? Now that you have aligned with your goals, it will be easier to rock the reflection. Consider these key questions regarding the situation:

1. List all the areas in your life where you are taking it personally. Where are you holding a grudge?
2. Ask yourself what you don't like about this situation or person.
3. How is that a reflection of you?
4. What can you learn from this situation?

Be compassionate with yourself and be open to receiving guidance.

∽

MOTIVATIONAL MANTRA

"What others say and do is not about me.
I release my need for others' approval
because I approve of myself."

FIFTEEN

Find Your Purpose and Passion

We feel like something is missing.

Nick Vujicic is an Australian motivational speaker who was born without any arms or legs. You can imagine the amount of bullying and ridicule he faced growing up, looking so different than everyone else. His entire life he felt different, but he also felt a deep disconnect from everyone around him. He had no idea what the future held for him. He didn't know that he was going to be on *Oprah*, or become a multi-book bestselling author, or become a motivational speaker spreading the message of hope to millions across the world, or have a beautiful wife and little boy. All he knew was that he had no arms and legs and that he was different. When he was young, he hated himself and was confused as to why he was here on earth. He was extremely depressed as a child and he didn't have hope. He tried to commit suicide by drowning himself. When we don't have hope we don't have the will to keep going.

I had the opportunity to see Nick speak live in front of a crowd of four thousand people in Maui, Hawaii. As he shared his personal story, he paraphrased Mark Twain and said, "There are the two most important days of your life: the day you are born and the day you find out what your purpose is. And if we don't know what our purpose is, it can be hard to know why we are alive." When Nick found his purpose, when he knew why he was alive, he no longer felt confused, angry, or disconnected.

Yes, we all have a deep desire to know our purpose, but I want to caution you: Too many of us get lost even further when we go searching for it. For many of us, we try so hard to find our purpose that we walk around feeling as if something is missing. Almost every single coaching client first comes to me with the desire to fill that void, to feel more, to stop going through the motions, the longing to find their purpose and tap into their passion. This notion that something is missing is a universal emotion that connects all humans. We are all looking for something, and we try to fill that void by reaching for things outside of ourselves—new clothes, new cars, vacations, relationships, and approval from others. Then when we get the thing we thought we wanted, we still feel that void. Why is something still missing?

This is how I felt when I was stuck in my corporate job, and I turned to drugs and food to try to mask the emptiness, to try to find what was missing. It wasn't until I got in touch with my passion and purpose did that empty feeling go away. For me, Nick Vujicic, and countless others who now know their purpose, the start of that journey was reaching for hope. Hope is the catalyst for removing that emptiness. **Hope is the bedrock of change.** If we don't have hope or we don't believe things can get any better, then we stay stuck in the empty void.

The challenge is that we don't really know what our purpose is until we find it. We have to trust that we will find our purpose even if we can't see it right now. If you only believe what you see, you can't get to where you want to go. Finding your purpose and passion is a lot like a road trip. If you have ever taken a trip across the country, then you know you have a destination, but you can't always see the entire path or way to get there. You drive along the road, and sometimes there is construction or detours that cause you to change course. You ultimately know you are on your way to the new destination, but the real journey is how you get there. So many of us feel a desperate need to have it figured out; we need to know our purpose, and because we don't, we feel something is missing. But we often gloss over the path that leads us to finding our purpose, which is unfortunate, for it is this path that leads us to ourselves.

The turning point for every person who has crossed over into living a life free of the void is the moment they start believing in something they can't see. We have to believe that our life can become better even if we don't see traces of it in our current reality. Instead of looking at what is not working, we have to learn how to aggressively push toward a better reality. This is the same for any situation in life where we want it to improve. If you are in an unhealthy relationship, you have to believe that you are deserving of and can be in a healthy, love-filled partnership. You hold your attention on what you want, not what is. If you are in a job you dislike, but you don't know what job would make you happy, you have to reach for the hope that there is something better for you. Feeling hopeless is the fastest way to kill our passion and prevent us from finding our purpose.

How do you find hope in hopeless situations? You turn to something bigger than yourself—a belief that there is a way out. You find inspiration to keep going by turning your attention to love instead of fear. You turn to trust!

When I very first left corporate, I had no idea what I wanted to do with my life. I just knew that corporate climbing was not for me. In fact, it was killing me. Once I left that work style behind, I made a choice to focus forward and to feel my way to happiness. This meant that I let go of thinking there was a right or wrong choice, and I followed the route that felt most joyful. In doing this I kept my eyes focused forward. Instead of focusing on what wasn't working, I chose to be thankful for what was. I found inspiration in people, places, and hobbies that fueled me with love. I trusted that I was going in the right direction. Within time, my true passion and purpose was revealed to me. Now I live every day on purpose and with passion. I made a choice to be in the journey of my life. I looked at finding my purpose and passion like the road trip. And each turn and detour led me to my dream job and life.

The same thing happened for Nick Vujicic. He said he used to look at other couples and feel jealous because he thought he would never have that. He didn't think anyone would love an armless and legless man. He knew he could never hold his bride's hand and he was angry at the world because it was unfair. His turning point came when instead of looking at the problem as the problem, he recognized that *the way he was looking at the problem* was, in fact, the only problem. His shift happened when he stopped praying for arms and legs and instead prayed with grace by thanking God for what he did have, a life. In Nick's lecture to the group, he said, "God never gave me arms and legs, but he healed my heart." Today he is married to a beautiful woman and they just had a baby boy and have plans for more children. He asked love to come into his heart. Once his heart was healed, he was able to have hope. And with that hope, he moved toward his passion to where he is today. The beautiful thing about this story too is it shows that we are only limited by our mind. Once Nick let go of his belief that he could never have a relationship with a woman because of his physical body, it happened for him. Believe in your purpose and it will come to you.

The truth is that your purpose is actually already inside of you; you have what it is you are looking for. Asking for love and being open to receiving it will help you experience life more fully and tap into the purpose inside.

The numb feeling that we all experience is because we feel disconnected from our purpose. One of the myths that keeps us feeling disconnected is the belief that our purpose is one specific thing—a job title, a relationship status, one specific role in life. But you are not a noun. You are more than just what you do. You are more than just one thing.

I had thought writing, lecturing, and sharing my message of happiness on playwiththeworld.com and in books was my purpose, but it wasn't until writing this book that I learned my purpose is to experience life.

Experience life! Live the full journey! **The purpose of life is to suck in the entire experience and love fully from the heart.** This is why we are here: to learn to grow and become more of who we are. And we can only do this by exploring, growing, and experiencing life in a variety of ways. Thinking there is only one specific purpose actually keeps you from reaching your passion-fueled life. The feeling that something is missing is because most of us don't give ourselves permission to follow through on all of our heart's true desires. We ignore the inner love nudge that says try this, explore that, and go experience this, and we hide out in our comfort zones as the feeling that something is missing grows.

One of my most popular group coaching workshops is the Find Your Purpose and Passion event. Every single person on earth wants to be happy, and we think if we know our purpose we will be happy. But I say you must find your passion first and *then* you will find your purpose. When you find and act on what you are drawn to, you love your life fully. Your purpose is to experience life, and you can do that by becoming more of who you really are.

Are you ready to find your purpose and passion? This is the most pivotal joy route of this book: accessing your heart so you can live your passion-filled life with purpose.

$\backsim$

JOY ROUTE
Find your purpose and passion.

When I first left my corporate job, I had a difficult time enjoying simple pleasures because I spent so much of my time focusing on what I was going to do next. What was my purpose? What was my passion? I spent enormous amounts of energy trying to figure out what I was supposed to do with my life. After a lot of tears, self-torture, and trial and error, I gracefully came to the realization that I couldn't think my way into my passion. You can't figure out your life purpose by thinking your way into it. It can only be felt in the heart. When we drop from our head—the frantic, trying-to-figure-it-out, and obsessing-because-we-haven't-yet-nailed-it head—to our heart, we energetically align with our joy; we become expansive and uplift the world because we are living in our light. The feeling that something is missing is replaced by love.

That empty feeling inside that we are all walking around with is a lack of love. Love can be God, Jesus, the universe, Buddha, or whatever you believe in. The point is, it is a love-filled presence that exists, and allowing that in is the key to embracing your purpose and passion. You are here to experience life fully. Your life passion is part of your purpose. When we deny ourselves joy and avoid acting on what makes us passion filled, we feel empty and lost inside. To fix this problem, we can start to put more joy in our life. The best method I found to do this is start with HOPE.

HOPE is used as an acronym in this joy route. As you go through each step, recognize that HOPE is the foundation for reaching your life's passion and purpose. When you do these steps, you will no longer feel as if something is missing. You will be full of love and light.

Awesome Action 1—H: Habitual Happiness

Awesome Action 2—O: Open Up to Optimism

Awesome Action 3—P: Purpose-Filled Passion

Awesome Action 4—E: Embrace the Journey

AWESOME ACTION 1—H: Habitual Happiness

The first step is to make our own happiness a habit. I know from personal experience that happiness is 100 percent a habit. I realized this when I left my corporate job to follow my heart and become a writer and life coach. In the process, I had to walk away from drug addiction and eating disorders, which prevented me from being happy. I had to learn new habits to support my happiness.

In order to embrace habits that support our happiness we need to recognize and unlearn habits that keep us from happiness. We all have barriers blacking us from bliss, and part of this joy route is to remove them. Unfortunately, many of these happiness-hindering habits are rooted in beliefs that society taught us were true.

Take a look at these twenty "truths" you should unlearn in order to be happy. As you go through the list, see which ones you identify with the most.

1. There Is a Right or Wrong Way to Do Something.

Trying new things and exploring different processes is part of growing. What works for one person may not work for you. Find your own process and your own beliefs, and let others have theirs.

2. Fitting in Is Belonging.

Trying to fit in means you have to contort yourself to fit other people's views. Doing so is not being true to yourself. Instead of trying to fit in, focus on aligning with your true self. You will belong when you are fully comfortable with yourself because you won't need others' approval.

3. Working Hard Will Make You Successful.

The harder you work, the more worn out you will be. You won't be able to fully enjoy your efforts. Instead of working harder, consider working smarter. Gauge your success by how much joy you are experiencing.

4. Failing Is Bad.

Failing is a fabulous way for you to learn more about yourself. When we try things and they don't work, it is an opportunity to figure out why it didn't work and how you can do it differently to succeed. The most successful people in the world have failed a million times. Ask yourself if you are failing enough.

5. Being Alone Means You Will Be Lonely.

When you enjoy your own company, you will find you are rarely ever lonely.

6. Life Is Supposed to Be Smooth and Free of Problems.

The ups and downs of life are how we live a balanced life. Embrace each turn and allow for the changes; you will feel peace when you stop resisting.

7. What People Think of You Should Be Important.

The only thing that matters is what you think about yourself. Work on your relationship with yourself, and you will feel more love and joy than you ever thought possible.

8. If You Were Skinnier, Prettier, or Smarter, You'd Be Happier.

Waiting for happiness to arrive based on a destination outside of yourself will keep you in a constant chase. How many times have you actually reached that goal weight, found that dream relationship, landed that so-called perfect job, and yet you still weren't happy? Every time! Happiness is not a place outside of us; it is inside of our own hearts.

9. Your Life Is Off Track.

Feeling like you are not where you are supposed to be or that your life hasn't turned out the way you planned keeps you from enjoying the present moment. You are right where you need to be. Trust that everything is in right order.

10. Letting Go Is Giving Up.

Letting go of stuff that weighs you down is the key to reaching new levels of success and happiness. When you let go of what no longer serves you, you stand up for yourself and realize you deserve better.

11. You Should Hold on to What You've Got, Because the Life You Know Is Better Than the One You Don't.

Learn to be comfortable with the unknown. We hold on to things that don't work because we fear the unknown and are afraid we don't deserve better.

12. You Need to Postpone Joy.

Retirement, vacation, and the weekend—all are excuses keeping you from enjoying life right now, in this moment. Reach for happiness every day and you will no longer need a vacation to achieve balance in your life.

13. You Should Listen to Your Head over Your Heart.

Your head will talk you out of what you feel is right. Trusting the guidance of your heart is never wrong. Ask yourself if the situation feels right, instead of thinking your way through the problem.

14. If You Don't Know How to Make It Happen, You Shouldn't Go for It.

We learn the way to achieve our dreams on the way to achieving them, so go for it. Your future self will thank you.

15. Unsupportive People Don't Care About You.

What others say and do has nothing to do with you. If you have a dream that people don't support, ask yourself if you believe in it. The more you believe in yourself and your dreams the less you need others to.

16. Self-Love Is Selfish.

When you show up for yourself, you can show up for the world.

17. Your Dreams Should Take a Backseat to Responsibility.

Your dreams *are* your responsibility. Don't let excuses keep you from following through on your purpose.

18. The Destination Is the Reward.

There is no destination; the journey is the reward, so start being present during your journey.

19. Being Vulnerable Is a Sign of Weakness.

Fully sharing yourself is the key to a happy life. Being vulnerable means you don't hide away; instead you fully embrace yourself and shine your light.

20. You Are What You Do.

You are not a noun. You are so much more than your job title, role, or position in life. Start celebrating you for you, because you make a difference just as you are.

It's time to pull out your joy journal and go inward to answer these powerful questions. Take a look at the list above and answer these guided questions.

1. What five society pressures do you fall back on the most? (Which do you identify with the most from this list? Write them down here.)

- _____

- _____

- _____

- _____

- _____

Now see how those habits have blocked you from being happy.

After looking at the habits blocking you, you can now cultivate more compassionate habits and make happiness a choice.

2. What ways can you make healthier mental choices when it comes to happiness?
3. Do you believe in your own happiness? Freewrite on this topic.

AWESOME ACTION 2—O: Open up to Optimism

Opening up to optimism is about focusing on the good instead of being resentful about the bad. Nick Vujicic was born without legs or arms. But today he is a world-renowned messenger of hope. He demonstrates that the only barriers in life are the ones we put on ourselves. We can choose to focus on our broken pieces and what is not working, or we can choose to see the good. We always have a choice. We can be angry for what we don't have, or we can be thankful for what we do have. Turning to the good will help you get out of your own way.

Regarding the situation causing you the most stress, focus on what is working! List out all the good things you are grateful for in your life.

AWESOME ACTION 3—P: Purpose-Filled Passion

Lose the idea that you have one purpose and are here to do only one thing. This thinking can block us from accessing what it is we are here to do, which is feel love, be love, and give love. Love shows up in many ways throughout our life. It is the romantic relationships; it is the cuddle session with your favorite furry friend; it is the walk barefoot on the beach, the swim in the ocean, the gardening, then eating fresh foods and nourishing green juice; love is joy.

What brings you joy? Every single one of us has our own inner joy route and things that feel loving to us. This awesome action is where you can get in touch with them. The more you open up to love, the more you will realize your true purpose and passion. The goal is to use your passion to live a purpose-filled life. Give yourself permission to be in the journey of life and explore your passions. Over the next thirty days, start to explore your passions. When you feel drawn to something, follow through on that inspiration. If you keep getting the idea to join a new fitness studio, take a cooking class, or study a new language, these are passions trying to poke through. Let yourself be guided by your passions. Do not put expectations on them; your only job is to follow them and allow them to guide you. Enjoy the process of living your passion.

What five passions will you explore in the next thirty days?

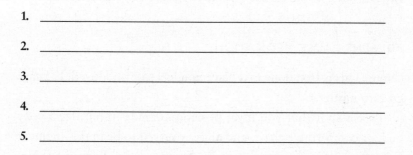

1. _____

2. _____

3. _____

4. _____

5. _____

Now pick one of these passions that speaks to you the most. In other words, which one are you most excited to pursue?

I am excited to pursue _____

What three actions steps can you take to move this passion into reality?

1. Action step 1: _____

2. Action step 2: _____

3. Action step 3: _____

AWESOME ACTION 4—E: Embrace the Journey

Just like a road trip, let yourself be in the journey of life. The journey is where the adventure is. The exploration is what will help you feel more fulfilled. The feeling that something is missing will disappear because you are embracing the journey and living with more passion. Let love guide you. Follow the route that feels loving and joyful. If it feels heavy and fearful, don't go that way. Always choose love. Let love pull you into happiness. You will discover your purpose-filled life by being present in the journey of life. In order to fully embrace the journey, you have to become present in it. Explore this meditation, which can help you release expectations of the future and be more present in the moment.

PRESENT PAUSE MEDITATION

(Note: This is best done in a place you feel safe and loved. I always go into nature.)

Pick a spot that you love, possibly outside in nature, a cozy bed, or comfortable chair, and allow yourself to be in this moment fully. Breathe in deeply with your eyes wide open. Focus on something close to you, like a tree, a leaf, or photo and look deeply at it. Study the colors. Explore its contrasting edges and textures. Take a deep breath in and touch the object. How does it feel? Does it feel the way you expected? How does it make you feel when you touch it? Was there a shift in your body when you reached out to touch it?

Now lean in to smell the object. Does it have a smell? Does that aroma remind you of another experience in your life? Does this object have a sound? Listen to the message of the object.

Now stay in this space of studying, analyzing, and loving the object for at least one more minute. This meditation is a way to help train yourself to be more present in everyday activities. We all crave love. We have a desire to be loved, give love and receive love. When you are present, it is a loving gift to yourself and to others. Cultivate more love by being present. This experience will help you reach your passion with more clarity and live your life with purpose.

MOTIVATIONAL MANTRA

"Love will show me the way.
I choose love."

BONUS RESOURCE

If you want to take this step deeper, download this guided audio meditation:

"Present Pause," from the *Adventures for Your Soul* meditation album. Available on iTunes, Amazon.com, or playwiththeworld.com/home/shop/

SIXTEEN

Be a Goal Digger

HABIT HINDERING HAPPINESS

We focus on what we don't want.

Are you where you want to be in life? Most people are not quite where they think they should be or where they really "want" to be. For the next chapter, let's just hang that mentality up for a while and recognize that you are EXACTLY where you are supposed to be. Consider that everything in your life that you have experienced has led you up to this point right here, right now. You have made no wrong turns, there are no mistakes, and where you sit, in this very moment, is perfect. What if you started to focus on what is going right instead of what is going wrong? This is a much better place to start from than feeling as if your life is off track, that you have made a wrong turn, or that you are not where you want to be. **Accept where you are fully to reach where you want to go faster.** You are not broken; there is nothing to fix.

If I were to ask you right now, "What do you want?" what would you say? When I ask most people this question, they will often tell me what they don't want first. *I don't want to work in this job anymore. I don't want to be single anymore. I don't want to have to worry about money.* Well that is all well and good, but my darling dearest, I asked, "What do you want?" You see, the majority of us spend so much time getting clear about what we don't like and don't want that we don't ever give ourselves time to think about what we actually want.

Take for example a common situation I often come across in my coaching sessions. Meet Samantha. She is someone who is ready to find love and meet a man that she can call her soul mate. She is on multiple dating sites. When she approaches social situations or plans to go out, she is often thinking about who she will meet, and asks herself, "Is tonight the night I meet my true love?" She will enter a room and scan the faces of strangers hoping to see a spark in someone's eye and a new potential match. When she doesn't have a love connection, she gets angry, maybe frustrated, and does not have as good of a time because her expectations were not met. She thinks thoughts like, "There are no good men left. Finding a stud is impossible when every man is a dud," and other harsh criticisms.

Samantha might read books on manifesting love, and feel as if she is doing everything right, but at the end of the day, after all her efforts, she still falls asleep alone and frustrated. Can you relate? She is trying so hard but her efforts are not met with her true desires. The trick here is to look at her efforts and focus deeper on what she is really doing. First, notice that Samantha is stuck in the "But Zone." She says things like: "I am ready for a relationship, but I don't think anyone will really like me for me," or "I want to meet my soul mate, but no one ever approaches me," and the old standby, "I want a relationship, but all the good men are taken." She is putting out a positive intention and then negating it.

Many of us do this, and it isn't just with relationships: "I want to leave my job, but I don't know what I want to do with my life" or "I want to lose weight, but everything I try doesn't work. I am hopeless." When we get caught in the "But Zone" we put our excuses, limiting beliefs, and fears in front of our desires. Naturally this prevents us from reaching our goals. For most of us we can't even get clear about our goals because we have so many "buts" kicking us in the face. Our excuses define our focus, and trying to move in a positive direction can become difficult.

The other thing that Samantha does is impose too many expectations. When she goes out, she wonders if that night will be *the* night she meets Mr. Wonderful. She is putting all of her hopes on one specific night. She's hoping that this one night will be the antidote for years of rejections, lonely nights, and failed relationships. She is putting her past into her present, and although she may think she is focusing on what she really wants, her desire is fueled by what she does not want—loneliness.

This is common; we focus on what we don't want in our life rather than focusing on what we really want. We do this because that is what we currently see in our life. It may feel challenging to move out of an experience that is so opposite of what you really desire. For example, Samantha wants to be in a loving relationship, but she keeps focusing on how she is single and alone. Her current reality of "what is"—being single—is contradicting "what she wants"—to be in a happy and healthy relationship.

The key is to focus on what you want despite what you have. If you want more money, instead of focusing on how little you have in your bank account, focus on the money you do have and the money you want. If you want to make a career move, instead of focusing on how miserable you are in your current position, think about the countless opportunities that are available to you. If you want to be in a relationship, don't focus on how undesirable you feel. Think about all the good qualities you have and show yourself some love. It is the best way to attract love. Using this method will help you attract anything you want. Love, abundance, health, and fulfillment.

Another good method to help you focus more on what you want is to surround yourself with people you admire and respect. Motivational speaker, author, and personal development king Jim Rohn said we are the sum of the five people we hang out with the most. Are you surrounded by negative gossip goal suckers or uplifting magic makers? When I left my corporate job, I left behind some friends as well. When I was depressed and addicted to drugs, my social circle was addicts and people who liked talking about their problems instead of trying to solve them. When I gathered up the courage to take a step forward toward finding my happy, I focused on where I wanted to be. I started to become friends with wellness bloggers, A-lister journalists, yogis, and *New York Times* bestselling authors. I felt more uplifted and started to see myself in a healthier light. My new social circle and the support they provided were invaluable in helping me move toward reaching happiness. Consider the five people you spend the most time with, and if you want to be in a different situation in your life, look at expanding your social circle to include more people aligned with your heart's true desire. If you want to be a six-figure income person, start hanging around people who make six figures. If you want to be athletic and fit, become friends with active folks.

Where we focus our attention is a significant factor in achieving what we want. Whether you want more love, more money, more freedom, or better health, whatever your desire is, it can come to you when you stop focusing on what is. "What is" is only temporary. It is a moment in time that is fleeting. Think about a time you changed your mind. Maybe you really wanted to join a club or organization, but after you thought about it more you realized it didn't fit your big picture. Maybe you were in a relationship with someone you loved, and then over time you realized you loved the person but were not *in love with* the person, so you went your separate ways. We change our minds all the time, from the moment we wake up, we might change our minds about how we want to style our hair, what clothes we want to wear, what route we take to work, what we want to eat. When you change your mind you are aligning with your true inner guide. Changing our mind is about aligning with what feels right in each moment. Naturally focusing on what feels good rather than what feels bad is the path to lasting happiness.

Samantha, our queen of looking for love, had already decided she will not be happy or have fun unless she meets "the one." There is nothing wrong with having hope; hope is a wonderful thing, but hope is not a strategy. We miss out on life when we focus on what is not here in the moment. Samantha wants to meet a man, but she is more focused on how he is not here yet. There is a big difference between *hoping* what you want will come to you and *knowing* it is on its way to you. Opt for *knowing*. When your heart and your head are aligned, you can release the expectations of "when" your desire happens, and you can relax into the journey more. Many of us focus so much on what we don't want because we don't trust or know that what we desire is on its way to us. There is a lack of belief fueling our current reality. If you are working toward a goal or dream, but you find it is taking a while to manifest, ask yourself if you believe it is going to happen. Get honest with yourself and really go inward to ask, "Do I believe this will happen for me?" There are many times when we spend a lot of time focusing on what we want with the best intentions of making our goals come true, but we don't actually believe they will come true. We don't always have faith in our worth. Samantha doesn't really believe she is lovable, and secretly feels she may be alone forever. Even though she wants to have true love, she is afraid it can't happen for her. Therefore it is easier to focus on what is not working and how she is still single than it is to try to muster up the courage to believe she is worth her desires.

If you are focusing on what you don't want more than what you do want, you will feel overwhelmed, stressed out, frustrated, and perhaps even depressed or sad. You may be feeling unhappy and hopeless. The goal is to turn your attention to what you want instead of what is at the moment, which requires a dedication to trusting the unknown. We can trust the unknown and become more comfortable when we follow the joy route of becoming a goal digger.

JOY ROUTE
Be a goal digger.

How do we retrain our brain to focus on what we want instead of what we currently experience? The answer lies in the dreamer inside your heart. Allowing yourself to dream will enable you to set goals and move toward achieving them. Goals are essential because they allow you to look ahead to where you want to go, instead of being stuck in where you are.

Some people don't set goals because they don't have a clear vision of what they want. They may say they want something—a new job, a new relationship, a leaner body—but they don't home in on what they *really* want. They don't have the specifics—what they are doing in the new job, the characteristics of their dream partner and how they feel in the relationship, what their healthy body looks and feels like. The key to having a clear vision is to imagine in detail what you want. Albert Einstein so eloquently said, "Imagination is more important than knowledge." Amen, bro, high fives to Mr. Einstein! If you can imagine it, you can make it become a reality. Call it visualization, call it dreaming, but we can't move toward something if we're not clear what it really is. We don't have to know how our goals will come true, but continuing to focus on what you want is much easier when you have goals to work toward.

You can't think your way into goal setting. Our mind has a way of censoring our dreams. *I would love to do that job, but it's impossible. I want to be in a relationship, but all the good ones are taken. I want to lose weight, but I have no willpower and will never succeed*. Instead, you have to imagine what you want and believe that you can have it. Your mind also has a way of being influenced. Well-meaning parents may try to convince you what career or course of study is best for you. With the best intentions, friends might try to convince you to take a certain path; if it's good for them, it must be good for you. But goals are unique to you, and only you. They are not for anyone else. So as we dive into this joy route, make sure you are aligning with your own desires and not being influenced by another's hopes for you.

Also recognize that goals change. What serves you at one point in your life can suddenly become restricting. Maybe you landed your dream job, and after a few years you realize you don't like the industry at all, or maybe you thought you met your soul mate but are no longer attracted to them. As you grow and circumstances change, your dreams can change and so too must your goals. Don't listen to your head, which may keep you in a situation that is no longer working. Drop into your heart to discover what you really want at the moment.

If you don't know exactly what you want right now because maybe you have been hanging out in the But Zone, or maybe you have been focusing so much on what you don't want that finding clarity feels like a fog, it's okay. These exercises can help. For me, in my own journey, I had no idea when I first left my corporate job that I would become a bestselling author, let alone even write a book. I didn't know I would become a travel writer or a life coach. In fact, I had no idea what a life coach was, and I certainly never saw myself as an inspirational speaker; I used to get sweaty and freeze up during presentations. But today, I can't imagine doing anything else. I have found my passion and purpose. Every day I do the work I love, and I fall deeper in love with it each day I do it. Falling in love with my life starts with becoming a goal digger. I had to set goals to get clear, remove my fear, and gain clarity into what I really wanted. And along the way, the more I explored and followed my heart, the more the goals came into focus.

Setting goals is an act of self-love. When you set goals, you are showing up for yourself and putting your desires into focus. It is a beautiful thing when you fall in love with the process of setting goals. This is the true essence of this joy route. Reaching your goals is only a minor fraction of the equation to happiness. Reaching your goals in fact is not the fun juicy stuff that keeps us fueled with passion.

Let's dive deeper for a moment. Pick a goal that you are working toward in your life. Maybe you want to lose twenty pounds, maybe you want to get married, maybe you want that sweet promotion your boss promised you. Now, imagine you wake up tomorrow and your goal is ACTUALIZED. Holy freaking awesome, you! Consider how it would feel if you woke up literally twenty pounds lighter, or next to the love of your life, or working from that corner office.

If you were to get really honest with yourself, it would be a little uncomfortable, and most people would not be up for the sudden change. We identify with ourselves on a daily basis with where we are in this moment in our life. And going without something to suddenly having it could be detrimental to the soul. This is why we hear stories of people who win the lottery and then go bankrupt, or people who lost all this weight and gained three times the amount back. Believe it or not, we actually need time to detach from the sense of self that is used to being in the current situation. Although we want change, pieces of us need to be released in order to move forward. There is a silent grieving process, but it can be a joyful one. Anytime you release something that no longer serves you, there is an artful dance of letting go. As we detach from the present state and step into our new state—whether it is losing weight, falling in love, or leaving a job for our dream career—we need to let go of our old self. It is necessary to honor the dance of letting go and trust the manifesting process.

I call this the universal buffer. This is the universe protecting us from wrecking our plan. We may think we know what is best for us, but the universe really knows what we need. This is why although setting goals is essential to having a joyful life, releasing the expectations around them coming true instantly is just as important as setting the goals themselves. I spent years trying to lose weight. My weight would fluctuate up and down, and although I thought I wanted the weight gone forever, waking up one day with all the weight gone would be unnerving. I wouldn't feel like myself. I spent years relating to myself with extra weight, that having what I thought I wanted instantly would be a striking contrast. The process of me losing weight over time is more natural and healthy. This letting go period is essential for manifesting our desires.

Our dreams are often big—and they should be. If your dreams don't scare you just a little bit, they're not big enough. But in order to achieve those dreams, we have to become the person who can sustain them. **Quick fixes are not the solution for long-term results.** For real, lasting results, we have to consistently move forward toward our dreams, gradually becoming the person we want to be. It's about consistent forward motion and dedication to the process.

Having our goal materialize instantly is not why we set goals; in fact, the journey to seeing our goal actualized is the real happiness trail. So for the moment, hang up the idea that reaching your goal is the magic pill to happiness, and give yourself permission to dance in the journey. Have fun trying new workouts and healthy food choices or impressing your boss in new ways. The pathway to reaching our goals is about following our joy, and when we follow joy we're living our life to its fullest. This is why the joy route isn't "reach your goals," it is to "become a goal digger." What is a goal digger? Goal diggers trust the unknown and use the journey for planning, dreaming, and doing. Goal diggers are happy, healthy, and always see the big picture. Goal diggers see opportunities when others see setbacks. Goal diggers know the power of saying no to opportunities that don't align with their true self, and they are confident with their choices. It takes a lot to bring a goal digger down, because they know that everything happens for a reason, and everything in life is happening for them, rather than to them. Goal diggers will compassionately consider all opportunities but lean on their gut instinct for life choices. Goal diggers are people who brighten up the room when they enter; they have a confident smile that radiates authenticity. They look inward to their own heart for answers. Goal diggers don't spend a lot of time worrying about the small things, because they recognize gossip, drama, and negativity will deter them from reaching their goals. Goal diggers dig deep inside themselves to access their own true voice, which creates an appetite for exploring life and learning about new things. Goal diggers set goals, and to others, it looks as if they are instantly manifested. They seem to have it all figured out, because goal diggers don't hang out in the negative space of what is, but rather the joyous place of what could be.

They focus their attention solely on what they want. Goal diggers make great friends because they show you what is possible. They don't preach their secrets to life, they simple practice what they are, and this is infectious energy that positively helps those around them. Goal diggers may set daily goals, weekly goals, and certainly monthly and yearly goals. They focus on big plans and work toward them. Every day, goal diggers focus on action toward living their ideal life. Goal diggers appreciate where they are, but thrive on learning and growing into more of who they are supposed to be. Goal diggers are freaking amazing!

Everyone can be a goal digger, but most people don't access that part of themselves because years of rejection, mistakes, and fear make it hard to move forward. But removing these barriers is what the activities in this book are all about. To help you become the best goal digger you can be, try this joy route in more detail.

AWESOME ACTION 1: Go on a Future Field Trip

This is a simple yet powerful exercise to help you access your authentic truth. This will support you in clarifying what will be important to include in your vision and goals.

Imagine Yourself in Five to Ten Years.
What are you doing? How do you feel? What does your life look like?

What Message Does Your Future Self Have for You?
Close your eyes and visualize yourself in one to three years. Ask your future self what message she has for you?

(If you want to take this step deeper, download this guided audio meditation: "Future Field Trip," from the *Adventures for*

Your Soul meditation album. Available on iTunes, Amazon.com, or playwiththeworld.com/home/shop/)

VISION BOARD YOUR LIFE.

Put your creative chops in action. A vision board is a collection of images, words, and ideas that inspire, motivate, and encourage you. Cut out pictures from magazines or that you find online, or, if you are feeling inspired and love to draw, sketch out images, words, and ideas that represent your ideal future. Have fun. Share your vision boards with friends and me; I'd love to see them. Use hashtag #Find-YourHappy on Instagram, Twitter, or Facebook. There is a power in sharing your goals with others; you are declaring on a deeper level "This is important to me," and your future self will thank you.

AWESOME ACTION 2: Dream on, Dreamer

Deep dive into your own heart to uncover what it is you really want for yourself. Give yourself permission to dream bigger and uncover your truth by answering these questions.

Get out your joy journal and whip up some fun answers.

1. If someone handed you an unlimited amount of money, what would you do with your day?
2. When are you the happiest? What are you doing, how do you feel?
3. If you had only six months to live, what would you do?
4. Visit your future self in five years. What is she/he doing? Who are you with? How do you feel?
5. When do you feel the most uplifted and joyful?
6. What is the thing you are best at? What is effortless and fun for you to do, share, and be? What is the sweet spot that gives you that uber-rush?

7. If you were to die tonight, what would you regret not doing?
8. If you could be known for one thing, what would it be?
9. When you were a young child, what did you love to do?
10. When do you feel the "there's a lot more where that came from" feeling?
11. When do you lose a sense of time because you are so engrossed in the moment?

After answering these questions, you will have clarity into who you really are and what brings you the most joy. You can then begin to craft goals that are grounded in powerful passion.

AWESOME ACTION 3: Become a Goal Digger

My Ideal Life:

Your goals and vision belong to you. You don't have to explain them or defend them to anyone. They are part of you and what you want to experience in life. Allow your heart to be your compass and dive in deeper with this ideal life exercise.

You'll know that you're heading in the right direction when you are excited and nervous reading it.

Your Vision:

- Is based on the idea that ANYTHING IS POSSIBLE
- Gets to the heart of your greatest ambition
- Supports you right now in making choices that lead you to your exciting future life
- Can be changed by you at any time
- Is personal; it is yours and not for anyone else. It is not what other people want for you. It is what you want for you.

Take some time to write, dream, and plan out your ideal life. The best way to become a goal digger is to just dive in. Even if you don't feel ready, just put pen to paper. After your prep work you have already done, now you can make smart, actionable goals. Create short-term and long-term goals for each category.

When you make goals, be clear, specific, and positive. Use the present tense for the most impact as well. For example, instead of saying "I want to write a book," craft the goal like this: "I am successfully celebrating the book advance of X amount of money for my book X."

Use "I am" instead of "I will." This triggers your brain's response to ignite movement in the direction of your goal. The truth is, your brain doesn't know the difference between what's real and imaginary. If I told you to close your eyes and imagine you are hiking on a snow-filled mountain with temperatures below zero, you would begin to feel cold. Similarly, if I said to imagine yourself by a fire, toasty and warm, your body would begin to warm up. When you focus on what you want and create a clear vision, it will manifest faster.

With my coaching clients and my own personal life, I have seen great results with setting three-month goals, one-year goals, and three- or five-year goals. Try it out here.

THREE-MONTH GOALS:

- Health/Body:
- Career:
- Personal:
- Legacy Contribution:
- Dreams/Play:
- Relationship/Family/Friends:

ONE-YEAR GOALS:

- Health/Body:
- Career:
- Personal:
- Legacy Contribution:
- Dreams/Play:
- Relationship/Family/Friends:

THREE- OR FIVE-YEAR GOALS:

- Health/Body:
- Career:
- Personal:
- Legacy Contribution:
- Dreams/Play:
- Relationship/Family/Friends:

MOTIVATIONAL MANTRA:

"I joyfully put my desires in motion.
All my dreams are coming true."

BONUS RESOURCE

If you want to take this step deeper, download this guided audio meditation:

"Future Field Trip," from the *Adventures for Your Soul* meditation album.
Available on iTunes, Amazon.com, or playwiththeworld.com/home/shop/

SEVENTEEN

Illustrate Your Illusion

◦~◦

HABIT HINDERING HAPPINESS
We resist change.

Change is as inevitable as rain in Kauai, Hawaii—the rainiest spot in the world—where it rains nine months out of the year. Both here in Hawaii and back in the Pacific Northwest where I am from, the rain is part of everyday life. Some of us locals just put on our stylish rain boots and splash around, while others stay home and complain about it. We know it is coming, we choose to live in some of the wettest locations in America, yet many locals act surprised when it arrives.

It reminds me of the way many of us act when change is pushed upon us. There are the changes we don't plan for: diseases, the sudden divorce, the unexpected layoff, death, and the surprises that always pop up when things seem to be smooth sailing. For most of us, change represents uncertainty, and with uncertainty comes insecurity and worry.

We should all expect change in life. The Dalai Lama, the master of living in the moment, even said that life is nothing *but* a transition, so things will always be changing. Yet, most people are uncomfortable with change.

At times, change can be magnificent. Especially when we choose to change, like the new makeover, new shiny car, the new fitness routine that makes us feel vibrant, we decide to have children, revamp our love life, we say yes to that dream promotion. These are the changes we welcome with a giant bear hug. But change is not always a joyful, happy time, but rather a grin-and-bear-it time. Your daughter is moving away to a different state for school or your live-in boyfriend of three years calls it quits, and now you are alone. That's what change seems to be for a lot of us—that stuff you have to plaster a smile over and pretend to embrace even when your heart is drowning in heartache.

The reality of change is that most of us want it as much as we are afraid of it. We say things like, "I am so unhappy in my marriage but I'm afraid of being alone," "I'm sick of working in corporate but I have no idea what else I would do," or "I can't stand where I live but my home is paid off." This is the But Zone; once again we fall into thinking things are bad, but the unknown is scary so we will settle for bad. The thing to remember is that all change actually happens *for us, not to us*. Whether it is change that is planned or life changes that seemingly happen for us, when change comes knocking on our door, it is the universe telling us to reexamine our life and consider what direction really matters most. **When we resist change, it is because we are still holding on to what the universe is asking us to release.**

Change is meant to get rid of old patterns, habits, situations, and people that no longer serve you. It is meant to be a new beginning. The pain comes when we hold on to what we are supposed to release. We are used to what is familiar and we often cling to what is safe and comfortable.

In my own life and working with coaching clients, I focus on getting past the fear of change and doing what we can to learn about the fear and why it is there. If we try to avoid our fear or turn a blind eye to it, it will ramp up because we are avoiding change's call and likely avoiding our heart's true desire. And then we fall into crippling addictions—hello, late-night binges on ice cream and potato chips—or we turn to alcohol, overworking, over-exercising, over-anything to escape the painful conflict of safety versus joy. Fear itself isn't a bad thing; it acts as a protection mechanism to keep us safe and secure. But fear arising when we are in transition or need to make a drastic life choice usually means our head is trying to keep us in the comfort zone.

One way to relax into change and stop resisting is to set more goals. And I know you are now a master at goal setting because you just learned all about how to become a goal digger in the previous chapter. Setting clear goals helps create a road map for us to follow when we find ourselves in unknown or uncertain territory.

The reality is, change is part of life. And the good news is, whether you like it or not, change is going to take place all the time, with or without your approval. The universe has a natural way of balancing things out, so even if you decide not to make any changes in your soul-sucking job, to that lousy relationship, or the painful conflict with your sibling, all of these things will change in time in a way that ultimately is in your best interest. But from my own experience and working with hundreds of clients going through change, it is much more enjoyable if you make change instead of waiting for the universe to do it for you. Still, some of us may take heart in the universe's relentlessness. Even if we do nothing, or are anxiety-ridden about the future, we can be assured the universe will sweep in and solve our problem naturally. (Personally, I would rather be proactive, rather than go kicking and screaming into change. It is a much more joyful route and truly an adventure for your soul.)

Take for example my own situation in preparation to move to Hawaii. I had one freelance writing and design client who was a local company based in Portland, Oregon. They loved having their freelancers in the same city; even though I worked from home, they liked the peace of mind of knowing their writer was in the same city. All of my other clients were thrilled about me moving my business to Hawaii, but I knew this company was not going to approve of it, but they were one of my largest clients. I spent months worrying, spending energy trying to figure out the best way to tell them, when to tell them, and scared of what would happen once I did. I worried myself into exhaustion, losing sleep and being distracted from anything else that was going on in my life. Four weeks before I was preparing to hop on my plane to Hawaii, I got a call from the owner of the company. He said they no longer needed my services. Now mind you, this was a significant amount of my income every week—about 60 percent. I had two choices: freak out and worry about my lost income stream, or see this as an answered prayer. I chose the latter. I knew right away that this was the universe doing for me what I couldn't do myself. Now I could go to Hawaii worry free and unchained to this client. For the next forty-eight hours, anytime my mind went to worry about what I was going to do about making money, I would instead say, "What do I want to happen?" And do you know what happened? Within forty-eight hours I got a book deal with one of the largest book publishers in the world. And I doubled my life-coaching business within three weeks. Miracles happen! When we take out the worry, they can manifest faster. Know that you are always being taken care of and trust things are working out in your favor.

When change happens, we can resist it or embrace it. You can make change from inspired action or desperate action. But even so, your only choice is to move forward according to what information you have right now. So many of us over-worry and trap ourselves into indecisiveness. This is a side effect of this emotional habit hindering our happiness. When we resist change, we often cling to things that no longer work for us. Naturally taking one step forward will help you feel more in control when change presents itself. Remember that small steps will reap large rewards when it comes to moving through transitions in your life.

Instead of resisting change, ask yourself why you are afraid to move forward. Is it because the path is unclear? Maybe you are scared to let go of something. Maybe you are not really ready to move on. Understanding our motivation for resisting change can help us embrace it more gracefully. The fear that drives you can help you understand your path. Don't negotiate with your fear. Just look at it for what it is: a sign alerting you that something different is on its way. If we don't have a plan for our life, we will often bash around in the uncomfortable transition. But when you create a solid plan for yourself, you have a big-picture focus that you can align with when change happens. This helps lessen the blow of all life changes and it also helps you find more peace. But we can't create a plan until we illustrate our illusions.

JOY ROUTE
Illustrate your illusion.

This joy route is paved with tools to help you align with your future self so you can be calm and cool through transitions. Instead of resisting change, you will begin to welcome it. Even though change happens all the time, when we are anticipating it, it can feel unnerving to just wait. Change can be difficult when we hold on to the past or when we are unclear of the future. If you are in the middle of transition, it can be difficult to navigate new territory. You might be mentally in the future but physically still releasing the past. Be kind to yourself through the transition. **The more present you are, the more successful you will be in your new situation.**

The last four years of my life have been a giant unfolding of change for me. I was forced to let go of who I thought I was in order to become who I really am. I walked away from a demanding corporate job in advertising, along with drug addictions, eating disorders, and a bad romance, to follow my heart and become a writer and life coach. I moved back to my hometown to get grounded and be close to family. But after four years, my restless heart began to stir and I craved a new change, which is one of the reasons I came to Hawaii to finish writing this book. We sometimes get to a point where change is mandatory because we have learned everything we need to in our current situation. Ask yourself if you are feeling restless, bored, or antsy. These are all side effects of staying in one situation too long. Relationships, jobs, and even places have built-in expiration dates. The resistance comes when we hold on to what the universe nudges us to let go of.

Through every transition, there is a delicate balance of holding on and letting go. We are releasing parts of us, but still growing into who we are supposed to become. When you think about changes, instead of resisting them, you can illustrate your illusion. An illusion is a thing that is wrongly perceived or misinterpreted by our senses. Most illusions are false creations in the mind that we lean into as real. Fact: Your boyfriend doesn't call you back. Illusion: You assume he is cheating, like your last boyfriend. Fact: Your boss doesn't say hi when he comes to work. Illusion: You assume this means he hates you. Illusions are shady because they will trick us into thinking they are real. When we lean into our illusions, they will run away with our fear; feeling fearful will amplify the illusion.

The idea of this joy route is to illustrate your illusion to disengage its detrimental abilities. By examining our illusions we can take a step back and see that the things we worry about the most are actually not anything to put extra energy into. Illusions separate us from love and keep us stuck in fear. The things we worry most about are illusions.

Our fear-based mind is always creating illusions that can sneak in and sabotage our efforts to be happy. To avoid self-sabotage through change, ask yourself these five essential questions.

1. **Am I running away from or to something?**

Ask yourself if you are running away from something or avoiding a situation by escaping it. "Am I feeling pushed or pulled?" When situations become unbearable, we often feel pushed up against a wall. We may feel trapped, stuck, or even paralyzed by the burdensome outcome. We may be looking to make a change because of desperation. These changes are usually scarier, unplanned, and emotionally exhausting, whereas feeling pulled by inspiration will help you make a more peaceful transition. To make real change last, choose to access your motivation from inspired actions; this will feel like a pull from your heart—joyful and full of love.

2. **Am I focusing on what I really want, or settling for what I think I can get?**

Always ask yourself, "Am I settling?" Many of us focus on what we think we can get, not what we actually want. If you want a raise, focus on the actual number you really want, not what you think the company will give you. **Don't expect the worst, plan for the best.** Most often we settle for less because of past mistakes that lead to outcomes we regret, which can fog up our rational thinking. We settle for what we think we can get because of the illusions and fear in our mind. We make choices based on past fears, which can prevent us from living more fully. Ask yourself what you really want, write it down, and focus your intentions on it.

3. Am I listening to others' opinions too much?

When we make life changes, whether they are inspired by ourselves or pressed upon us, we may lean on friends and family for support. What other people tell you about your situation is a reflection of them and their own life experience, fears, and past choices.

It is great to listen to others, but wise to ignore them. You, yourself, know in your heart what is best for you. Other people do not have your perspective or big picture in mind. Most people try to help, but when we listen to them we can drown in lack of clarity. Do yourself a favor and check in with yourself instead. Ask yourself the questions you would ask a friend. The first answer that comes to you is usually your inner guide talking to you. Trust that inner voice. Ask yourself, "Do I trust myself?" and take steps to cultivate a healthy relationship with your gut feelings.

4. Does this choice feel expansive or restrictive?

When we make choices based on fear, they will feel heavy and burdensome. When you make your choices based on inspiration and hope, they often feel expansive and joyful. Choose the joyful, love-filled route. Your choice will be more rewarding, and you will have no regrets.

5. Am I holding on to things I can let go of?

One of the side effects of life changes is a growing pain. All change requires growth, and if we hold on to our past, it can prevent us from moving forward. All change represents a new period of our life where we can welcome in new opportunities. If we hold on to too many things, beliefs, physical stuff, and emotional burdens, we will not have room for the new goodness to come in.

Use the transition time to strip down, de-clutter and remove things, thoughts, and relationships that you don't want to carry into the new period. We often hold on to things that no longer serve us out of fear of losing what we worked so hard for. Do your future self a favor and get rid of it. You know what "it" is. If you are even having doubts about it, it is time to release it for good. We have to let go of the junk that weighs us down so we can fly.

Let's take it deeper. Try these awesome actions out to truly break the habit of resisting change.

AWESOME ACTION 1: Surrender

"Surrender" is a disturbing word for a lot of people. It sometimes feels passive or like we are being asked to give up. But surrender is actually aligning ourselves wisely with what is beyond our control. Life changes like getting older, losing a furry friend, and getting sick are all beyond our control. You can choose to be angry or resentful at life, or accept it. Surrender is not saying, "This is okay. I give up." It is accepting that some things are truly out of your control, which means putting faith into divine timing and trusting that the universe has a plan greater than yours. My friend Gabrielle Bernstein always says the universe has got your back. All you have to do is trust that things are working out for you, not to you.

> *"If we are facing in the right direction, all we have to do is keep on walking."*
>
> —PROVERB

We try to control things because we fear what will happen if we don't. The irony is that attempting to control situations actually makes us feel *less* in control. We're trying to harness something that can't be stopped, and that makes us feel helpless. Trying to control things is also counterproductive because if you are micromanaging details or obsessing about the future, you're blocking necessary change. The relentless universe will just work harder to accomplish what needs to be done.

> Surrender
> = 100 percent acceptance of what is
> + Faith that all is in right order

Surrender is not about sitting on your butt and doing nothing. It's about taking thoughtful action from a place of trust. Know that letting go of control and surrendering fully not only feels better, but actually will produce better results. For most of us, it's to make the shift from control to surrender. Here are some questions that can guide you:

1. If I let go of control, what am I afraid will happen?
2. Would letting go feel like freedom?

When I ask coaching clients these questions, they are able to get out of their own way. The second question is extremely powerful because every time letting go does feel like expansive freedom, they know it is the right thing to do. Freedom is what we all want. The real resistance comes because we aren't allowing ourselves to feel free, which is a natural human desire. We deny ourselves our own natural essence.

Surrender is acknowledging the change. When you do this you will feel more in control.

AWESOME ACTION 2: Designate No Worry Time

If you are going through a change, set aside time each day that is NO WORRY TIME. This means you don't worry about the future. Instead you focus on creating a solid plan to help you align with your highest good. Instead of focusing your energy on what "could happen," focus on what you *want* to happen. Pull out your joy journal and write a happy ending to any scenario that is currently troubling you. You can do a freewrite, or just jot down key phrases aligned with your goal. This no worry time can be a chunk of time every night, a two- to three-hour window where you actually develop a clear plan to move your dreams forward. When worry creeps in, you smack it down and say this is a no worry time. When you are flowing in this space, your ideas will feel fresh, you will be inspired, and be more motivated to take action. This no worry time can start small; if you are overwhelmed with fear and worry, take small steps and just set aside thirty minutes of no worry time. Say to yourself, "I won't worry. I will trust that things are taken care of." Then as you practice this, the time frame for no worrying will increase, and pretty soon you will be leaving a no worry life.

AWESOME ACTION 3: Illustrate Your Illusion

Albert Einstein said, "The most important decision we make is whether we believe we live in a friendly or hostile universe."

What are you beliefs about the world?

What are your beliefs about the transition and change you are going through?

Being receptive to life and allowing things to happen is a skill that you can cultivate. When you practice looking at your illusions and illustrating them, you will feel more relaxed into all chapters of your life.

I will tell you from personal experience and working with thousands of people in workshops, coaching, and lectures, that it helps to believe in a friendly universe—a place where you are supported and loved. When you feel the world is out to get you, you are combative, self-destructive, and fearful. To dive deep into your change, ask yourself what your beliefs are about the situation, and answer honestly. Then find the good ones and hold them near. There are always good beliefs; by nature we are hopeful creatures. We just need to tap into that hope and recondition our mind to focus on it.

Look at the illusions in your mind and ask, "Does this feel real?" We can always choose to embrace change and look at setbacks as growth. When you illustrate your illusions, you will flow through life with confidence and clarity. Enjoy your new awareness and awesome acceptance of life.

⁓

MOTIVATIONAL MANTRA

"All change is part of a greater plan.
I trust my life is unfolding perfectly."

EIGHTEEN

Sweet Surrender

HABIT HINDERING HAPPINESS
Destination disaster;
we think our life is off track.

We often worry that we have somehow gotten off course. We think that perhaps our life is off track, and we have made mistakes that are unfixable. Maybe you worry that you aren't quite where you think you should be, whether it is the job you thought you'd have by this age, the relationship status, or where you would be living at this time in your life. If you aren't where you thought you'd be, you may feel like a failure. I call this destination disaster, the feeling that our life is off track. This never-ending cycle keeps us constantly reaching for expectations that we have placed upon ourselves. These expectations are usually derived from unmet needs, and our mind tells us this is what we must do, be, accomplish in order to be fulfilled. If, for any reason, life doesn't go along with our plans, we take the blame and feel like a failure.

Western culture especially plays into this idea that you have to be somewhere or someone you aren't in order to be happy. Mainstream media is a big culprit supporting this idea that you are not where you should be in life, because it is a marketing master maven trying to keep people hooked into the idea that there is always more to have, do, or be. That's how they make money, after all.

Since moving to Hawaii, I have seen a shift in both my spending habits and my focus. I love being here because the Aloha spirit is about connection and embracing the moment. Material items are less important here, and the need to keep up with others is replaced by celebrating each other for who they are. This spirit suits me well. On the mainland and in many Western cultures the need to go, go, go is a cultural pressure. The need to be more, have more, spend more is a pressure that works its way into the cracks of our psyche. If we're not keeping up, we're falling behind.

Now before I lose you, this chapter is not about advertising and mass media, but it is important to touch on this significant topic in order to break up with this habit hindering our happiness.

I know firsthand about the powers of advertising and its effect on our culture. I spent years climbing the corporate ladder working at one of the largest advertising agencies in the world. As I designed billboards, television commercials, and print ads for some of the most powerful and profitable corporations, I learned the art of putting your best foot forward and showing only what you want the viewer to see. I spent hours on location with beautiful models, celebrities, and industry experts, art directing the shoot for the photographer to capture the perfect angle, the perfect shot, the perfect moment in order to manipulate the viewer into believing they "must" have a product. For example, did you know that a high camera angle looking down (even slightly) on a model would always make her appear more slender? These small nuances help create a feeling and a message to influence the average consumer. And when we have thousands of images, concepts, and points of view bombarding us every day, it becomes difficult to know which way we should go.

I suffered immensely when I worked in advertising, in large part because it wasn't what my heart was called to do, but also I didn't like that my job was to tell people how they should behave, or what they should buy, in order for them to feel good about themselves. Selling folks products in order to make them feel like their life was better didn't sit well with me. I am not at all saying that adverting is bad or a bad profession; I still have some great friends in the business and I teach marketing classes at the Art Institute of Portland to college students, but the corporate aspect just wasn't for me. And I do think many people are unaware of the subconscious effects advertising and media play into our decision-making process. Many of us feel like our life is off track because we have expectations set forth that we are not meeting. We fail to meet them in part because they are unrealistic. Carefully composed images, Photoshop, and manufactured moments are not real life. Trying to emulate these ideals is just setting everyone up for failure. Also, many times, these expectations go against what we feel is right for us. If you feel this inner conflict, it may be a hint that your life is really off track, and that you know in your heart a better path to take. Our hearts always know what is right for us. As long as we look outside of ourselves, we will never find our true selves or the happiness we really need.

When I was working in corporate, I felt like my life was off track. I was $70,000 in debt from putting myself through a graphic design program to be in an industry I thought I wanted but hated once I stepped into it, and all I had to show for it was a depressed life. It wasn't until I accepted what was and surrendered to my life not going according to my initial plan that I was able to make room for the life I was supposed to lead. When we let go of what we *think* we should do and exchange our control for trust, we begin to create space for miracles to enter. By letting go of the idea that I was supposed to run my own advertising agency by the time I was thirty, I was able to surrender to the plan the universe had for me—which is speaking, writing, and coaching. I am so much more connected to my work today, but I had to let go of the idea that I thought my life was off track in order to get here. Everything I went though was essential to help me do the work I do today. I lead from a place of truth and integrity, and my depression and experience in corporate help me connect to others. Trust that what you are going through right now in your life, even if you feel as if you are off course, is actually part of your bigger picture. The universe always has a plan greater than yours, and it is your opportunity to surrender to that.

When I was in high school, I tried out for the dance team. I had dreams of being a dancer, but when I didn't make the cut for the team I was devastated. I felt like my life was off track and I had failed. My mother told me, "It is this or something better." She used to always say that when I felt rejected. I later learned that all rejection is simple projection. Meaning if we don't get the position on the dance team or we don't get the job we think we want or the person we are into doesn't call us back, it is the universe's way of protecting us and keeping us open for something better. And something better is always around the corner. All we need to do is trust. If I made the dance team, I would have never had time to write for the school newspaper and be on the yearbook staff, and if I never did that, I wouldn't have found my love of writing and pursued a journalism degree. The universe has a big plan for you; get out of your own way, and realize everything you are going through is part of a bigger plan.

It comes down to this, when you let go of who you THINK you are supposed to be, the universe can swoop in and help you become who you are really MEANT to be. If you feel like you are off track and constantly playing catch-up to some ideal set forth for your life, the best thing to do is Sweet Surrender.

JOY ROUTE
Sweet surrender.

This joyful approach to breaking this habit hindering happiness is all about surrendering to what is and having faith in what will be. I will take you through steps to help you relax into the rhythm of your life.

Have you ever noticed that happy people have a certain spring in their step? They seem to walk their talk and illuminate the room as they shine with joy. Happy people seem to have figured out the heartfelt way to live a full life. Happy people have certain habits that keep them happy. I have learned that it comes back to habits. Everything we have done together so far is about breaking habits hindering happiness and making healthy emotional habits. In this joy route we're going to cultivate new habits that enable us to surrender to what is and trust in what will be.

AWESOME ACTION 1: Find the Silver Lining

It is important to look closely at your own life and consider where you feel off track. Ask yourself, what area of your life could be going better?

Now take a moment to reflect on past experiences and what may have felt like a setback, and actually turned out better than you planned.

List three disappointments in your life and then what the silver lining was.

Remember, when one door closes another opens, and often it is better than we ever thought.

Now return to the area of your life that feels off track, and ask yourself what the silver lining might be.

AWESOME ACTION 2: Avoid Mistake Hangovers

Mistake hangovers are a crippling way we stay trapped in feeling as if our life is off track. Avoid this destination disaster by looking at the areas of your life where you are holding on to regret. Regrets in life are most often unexplored opportunities where we wish the outcome were different than it really was. If you find that your mind often wanders to the past and what went wrong in certain situations, then you have a form of mistake hangovers. In order to clear space to allow your life to unfold naturally, answer these key questions.

1. What mistake are you holding on to?
    * Practice this meditation to help you remove the burden of this mistake. (If you want to take this step deeper, download this guided audio meditation: "Avoid Mistake Hangovers," from the *Adventures for Your Soul* meditation album. Available on iTunes, Amazon.com, or playwiththeworld .com/home/shop/)

    "Avoid Mistake Hangovers" Meditation
    Place your hand on your heart, and close your eyes and go inward into the situation that is causing you the most regret. Think about the mistake you feel you have made and allow yourself to sit and be present with it. Take a look at all the people involved in this scenario and imagine yourself in their shoes. What if what you think happened was only one part of

the entire picture. As you see yourself in the other person's shoes, imagine yourself standing across from them. You see yourself looking into their eyes. Send love to yourself and allow yourself to be fully present in this moment. Repeat these words: "There are no mistakes, there is only growth. I did the best I could with what I knew at the time. My story is unfolding perfectly and this situation happened to help me learn and grow into more of who I am supposed to be. I want a deeper connection to those around me and that can only happen when I release my past. I forgive the situation and I trust that all is in right order. I hand over this troubling time to the universe and I let the situation heal. I have made no mistakes, I have only learned more about myself, and that is the gift of this experience. I trust that all is in right order."

AWESOME ACTION 3: Sweet Surrender

Surrender is not giving up or saying that everything is perfectly okay; it is the willingness to let yourself energetically off the hook of trying to control the outcome. It is exhausting to try to be in charge all the time, which is why Sweet Surrender is your key to happiness. Surrendering is recognizing and accepting what you can't change. We do this by releasing expectations.

We try to control our life because of what we think is going to happen if we don't; basically, our control is sourced from fear. Control is the result of being attached to a specific outcome—one we are certain is the best for us. I often say when we try to control a situation we are trying to play God. When we are attached to the outcome, the universe cannot come in and help give us what we really need. Here's the deal: The energy behind surrender accomplishes so much more than the desperate energy of control. Think about the difference between the two. Control energy is tight, restricted, and often manic. Your mind may shift from the past to the future very quickly as you try to figure out the solution. Now switch to surrender mode; you are calm, peaceful, and connected to your truest self. You are more present in the moment and you can feel there are things happening behind the scenes to help support your desires and needs. You trust. You let go of the attachment by being present in this moment. If you are obsessing and micromanaging all the details of your life, you can guarantee you are in your own way. Step into the Sweet Surrender by going inward and repeating this mantra.

MOTIVATIONAL MANTRA

"I allow my life to unfold naturally.
I trust all is in right order.
The universe supports my desires and me."

BONUS RESOURCE

If you want to take this step deeper, download this guided audio meditation:

"Avoid Mistake Hangovers," from the *Adventures for Your Soul* meditation album. Available on iTunes, Amazon.com, or playwiththeworld.com/home/shop/

NINETEEN

Laser Your Inner Light

∾

HABIT HINDERING HAPPINESS
We think unsupportive people
don't care about our goals.

When I first started my business as a writer, life coach, and speaker, I struggled with feeling accepted by my friends and family. I felt like they didn't understand or support Play With The World. It seemed as if they didn't know this was a business and my future plan for my life. I felt so hurt when they didn't show up for my workshops, or read my newsletter. I struggled so much. I kept thinking they didn't understand me, or care about what I was up to. I recall the night of my very first public workshop when my dad said, "Are you sure you want to do this?" I felt like he energetically punched me in the gut. How could he ask such a crazy question? This is my heart and soul poured into this work. Yes, you bet, I want to teach people about happiness! Today the support from my family has shifted. Just last week I spoke in front of fifty people

at a self-love benefit I hosted, and my dad attended the lecture. It
was the second lecture he attended in four years. Afterward he
was blown away and said, "You are an excellent public speaker!
You can help so many people with your message. I am so proud
of you." A big difference from the unsure him many years ago.
The reason I share this story is that this chapter is all about helping you gain the confidence you need to pursue your goals, even
when people aren't supportive. Because in the end, what matters
is that you keep going no matter what. Because most often, when
you give yourself the support you want and believe in yourself, in
time others will come around, just like my father did.

But that doesn't mean when we are starting out on new dreams
and directions in life it doesn't hurt when people we love don't
seem to support our vision. What I didn't realize at the time was
that my father was really just asking me what I was afraid to ask
myself. Putting yourself out into the world is a scary thing. My
subconscious kept saying, "Are you sure you want to do this? What
if no one comes? What if this is a big mistake?" The lack of support I felt from my family and friends was really just a reflection
of my lack of belief in myself. Starting a new business or working
toward new goals takes courage, and most of the time we don't
really know if we can do it. We just have to go out and do what
we feel is best. So workshop after workshop, I put myself out there,
and within time my confidence grew. And no surprise, so did the
support around me. Today, my family is my biggest supporter,
attending my group coaching sessions, sharing my messages on
social media, and telling me how much they love what I am up to.

When you believe in yourself and have confidence, the rest of
the world will too. But it has to start with you. If you are in a
position where you feel like those around you are not supporting
you, the best thing to do is turn inward and asks yourself, "Do I

believe in myself?" Often we seek validation from others when we lack the belief in ourselves.

Naturally we want support, but stepping out of our comfort zone requires risk, and risk can be intimidating. In an effort to lessen the risk, we often focus our attention on the support of others. When those around react less than supportively, we take it personally and feel as if they don't care about us. At least this is what I experienced, and many of my coaching clients tell me they struggle with this often. When we start to move toward our dreams and pursue new goals, often those around us are not as enthusiastic. When our enthusiasm is met with nonchalant responses, we can sometimes become angry. This anger turns into resentment, and then we can easily fall into thinking, "The world is out to get me, nobody likes me." Then in the worst-case situation we even fall victim to the fear already inside our heads, and abandon our dreams. We think things like, "If nobody cares why should I even keep going?" And ultimately we give up before our dream has a chance to see the rewards of following through. All because we think unsupportive people don't care about our goals and therefore they don't care about us. The best way to combat this emotional habit hindering happiness is to recognize that it is fear, once again, in the driver's seat of your life. Anytime we look outside of ourselves, we are detached from authentic self. Instead of looking at what others are not giving you, look at what you are not giving yourself.

Recognize that when we begin to action out our goals, there is a giant energetic leap forward in the sense that we are putting enormous focus on what we want instead of staying where we are. This takes courage. When we are afraid of this leap, we desperately seek support from others to bolster us. Confidence is the great enabler that can help you stop focusing on needing support from those around you. But confidence only comes from action, so the more action you take, the more confident you will be. This is exactly what I started to do in my own business and with time, things transformed.

If you are spending your time thinking about why you aren't getting support from loved ones, instead start putting that energy into the goal. You waste time wondering why others are not there for you, and in doing this you are not there for yourself. You don't show up for yourself at the time you need yourself the most. So the natural fix is to show up for you. As you start taking more steps and moving toward your dreams, you can also recognize that your goals are for you. They do not belong to anyone else. When we want others to get on board with our dreams, we can often hinder our own ability to manifest our dreams. It sure does help to have supportive people around you, but if you are not supporting yourself, then others cannot show up for you either.

The turning point for me was recognizing that just because my close friends and family were not supporting my coaching and writing yet didn't mean they didn't love me. In fact it had nothing to do with their relationship to me. They all had their own lives and were busy living them. They loved me and supported me in the sense that they were happy I was happy, but asking people to be there for me when I wasn't even sure what I was doing was a tall order to ask for. The switch for me happened when I took all the energy I was wasting on feeling like my family didn't believe in me and turned it inward on believing in myself. Soon enough, I was invited to be on morning shows and share my message of happiness. International newspapers and radio shows contacted me to be in their outlets. The less I focused on others' support and turned my attention inward toward believing in my goal, the more I focused all my energy on making that a reality, the more opportunities came my way.

Instead of thinking unsupportive people don't care about you or your goals, laser your inner light.

~

JOY ROUTE
Laser your inner light.

Laser your inner light is all about connecting with your true essence. We can do this by getting to the "why." *Why are you doing what you are doing?* When you get in touch with the why, you can laser focus your attention on it. For example, one of my best friends is a fantastic artist. She does paintings that transform the viewers; there is so much love in her art that it is hard not to feel the love emanating off the canvas. Not too long ago, she had a gallery showing at a premier New York art gallery. She was very excited, but also told me she was concerned about money and selling her paintings. She was also unsure of the support she would receive. She knew her parents would come, but wasn't sure which friends would show up to the event. This uneasy feeling was blocking her from enjoying the process of seeing her art on gallery walls. I suggested she stop focusing on the money and instead get back to the "why"—why she paints. She loves painting and it is fuel for her heart. She lights up when she gets to share her art with the world, and when she is painting, it is not about money at all. Instead, it is about expressing herself and sharing her truth in gorgeous art. Her paintings touch the soul, and she is able to empower, uplift, and inspire people who look at her art. Her why is about healing and connection.

When we take our attention off what is not happening and instead focus on why we do what we do, we laser our inner light. Lasering your inner light is about connecting with your true essence and letting that be the driving force fueling your dreams.

When we do what we love from a place of passion, the support and money will always follow. But when we are looking for support and money first, it blocks the energetic flow of manifestation; we have cut the cord and stopped the flow of energy to our dreams. If you want to feel support and love for your goals, first give it to yourself. Put your energy into believing in your goals. You can do this by getting in touch with the why. When you laser your inner light, this becomes an infectious source of passion that others want to be a part of. When you show up fully, the rest of the world will too. But it always starts with you.

Once you get in touch with your why, the next best step is to take action by doing it now. This means have a sense of urgency with your dreams; do not wait until the time is right to take steps to make your goals come true. In order to feel support from others, we have to get honest with ourselves about why we are doing what we want support with. It might be frightening to take the first step that leads you to your dreams, but drop into your heart and find the confidence to do what you love.

Know that the confidence can only come with action, and the more action you take, the more you will learn and grow and the more empowered you will be. I didn't know I was going to be a public speaker; I just had a message to share and trained myself how to speak in front of strangers. Even now, I still have moments of insecurities and worry. Sometimes when I speak to new groups, my confidence wavers. When it comes to speaking to strangers, I find I am more comfortable when I speak to individuals in the group first. Many of the events I lead are in social groups, organizations, and wellness centers. When I arrive early to meet and greet the people attending, I feel connected and inspired. I get to know my audience and this always calms my nerves. However, on some occasions, I am on a large stage, and I am asked to stay behind the scenes until my name is called to present. Anytime this happens I feel rushed and nervous at first. So I learned that arriving early to meet the organizer and staff or mingle with people in the audience is a great way for me to make the connection I am craving. I have made it a habit to connect with people no matter what before I open my mouth to share my message. I found what works for me, and this may go against a traditional public speaker's approach. I know my friend Gabrielle Bernstein has a specific process of meditation before she goes on stage. This works wonderfully for her. The important thing is to find what works for you. Each person has their own way of getting confident. Lasering your inner light is about connecting to that inspiration inside and trusting yourself enough to know how to tap into it.

Connecting with my audience before an event is something I learned by getting out and doing it. I have hundreds of emails from people I met at events who were blown away by my openness and accessibility. This helps people feel like I am their partner on the journey to happiness. I even have people who have reached out and are super surprised at both my quick response and that I respond and not my assistant. I have made it a business practice to be accessible, because this works for me. I love connecting with people and helping others find their happy. I found what works for me because I lasered my inner light. Instead of focusing on the lack of support in my life, I shined my inner light, and now I have emails and support from people all around the world showing their love and support for the work I do.

Doing what works for you and honoring that it is the right path for you is essential to growing your confidence. Don't worry about what others do; the goal is to find a process that works for you. And it comes back to you finding out what you need to help you feel more confident. Ask yourself, "What do I need to feel confident?" You can only learn what your needs are through trial and error. Give yourself time to learn what works for you. This is an important part of the process, and as you learn more about yourself take mental notes. These little mental moments can help you feel more confident. Try it out for yourself.

AWESOME ACTION 1: Get in Touch with Your Why

Do you have a goal or dream that you are working toward but feel like those around you are unsupportive?

Get in touch with the why of your goal.

Why did you set out to achieve this goal?

Let the why drive your actions. It is about sharing your true self with the world and letting your passion guide you. Use that to emanate your why to the world. This will give you more support and success than focusing on why others aren't supporting you. Shine your inner light by aligning with your why. When you believe in yourself, you don't need others to believe in you. The best support comes from within.

AWESOME ACTION 2: Do It Now

Action out your goal! In order to get over the insecurities of starting something new, you must take action. What three things can you do today to work your dream into reality? Ask this every day. Always ask yourself, "What three things can I do today that my future self will hug me for?" Can you start a newsletter for your blog? Can you call a contact that a friend gave you to network? Can you hire a life coach or reach out to an author who has helped you? Can you pitch your article to the local newspaper? Have fun playing with action steps. Not all of them reap results, but all of your actions together will reap tremendous results. The more you do, the more you will flourish.

AWESOME ACTION 3: Laser Your Inner Light

A great way to stay focused on your goals is to connect with your inner light and laser it into everything you do. When you take action steps toward your goal, flood them with light. Literally imagine yourself full of love and light and connecting each action step to the highest good. It is like my friend who was at first worried about her gallery show and selling enough pieces to make ends meet. She was disconnected from her inner light. It wasn't until she flooded the evening with love and light that she felt supported, loved, and cared for. The universe will always support your desires when you are aligned with your true, authentic connection. Flood your desires and dreams with light, and with every action step, conversation, or outward expression ground it in love and light. Lasering your inner light is the fastest way to get over others not supporting you. You will be so connected to your true self that others can't help but to get on board with your dreams. You will illuminate the world, and this energy is infectious.

Once I put these practices into play, the support I longed for was front and center. The moment I realized the support was when I gift wrapped a copy of my first book, *Find Your Happy*, and put it under the Christmas tree. When my dad and mom opened up their signed copy, I saw tears in my dad's eyes. He was so proud and happy for me. There in his hands was the real full book I had been working on for so many months. Sometimes support comes to us in ways we don't recognize. Just because my dad didn't physically come to my events and he asked tough questions that pushed my buttons, doesn't mean he didn't care. I had never seen my dad cry; that moment touched my heart dearly and that is the moment it all sunk in. Just because others don't always show us support for our goals, it doesn't mean they don't love us. They support us energetically because ultimately when you surround yourself with supportive, loving people, the only thing they really want is for you to be happy. So focus on making yourself happy, and when you do, the support will flood in.

MOTIVATIONAL MANTRA

"When you believe in yourself,
other opinions don't matter.
The best support comes from within."

TWENTY

Let Go

HABIT HINDERING HAPPINESS
We are addicted to stress.

My dear friend Kristine Carlson, who so awesomely agreed to write the foreword of this book, has been through some turbulent times. Her late husband, Richard Carlson, author of the bestselling book series *Don't Sweat the Small Stuff,* said, "Stress is nothing more than a socially acceptable form of mental illness." Kristine is a fabulous example of not sweating the small stuff because she makes a conscious choice to live the big stuff. For many of us this idea sounds nice, but it is hard to practice when life drama arises.

Stress is something most of us can identify with on a daily basis. When is the last time you said you were too busy or that you didn't have time to do something because you were so stressed out? It probably hasn't been too long, because many of us often identify with one another through our stress. Our stress becomes a rite of passage into adulthood. We identify how busy we are with how stressed out we feel. Running the kids to school, attending the PTA meetings, making sure we get our Zumba and yoga time in; all that on top of ensuring the family is well fed and all the bills are paid! It is no wonder that stress has become the common currency of social acceptance. If you aren't stressed like the rest of the crazed world, working really hard to balance everything, then something must be wrong with you! When we look a little deeper though, we see that this is just a silly habit that keeps us from happiness.

When I work with new clients in my life-coaching and mentorship programs, I ask them their level of stress. Most people identify their well-being and happiness with low amounts of stress, but almost everyone shares stress levels that are very high, so by definition, this means they aren't happy. The things they are stressed out about range widely from worries about financial stability, being overworked, and exhaustion, to lack of clarity about their romantic life or career path. The things we worry about can eat us alive, but I have come to understand that stress is a common thread that connects us all. No matter the source of stress, we believe that stress is a bad thing, and yet we can't seem to break free from it. It is like an addiction.

Stress is a reaction to a stimulus that disturbs our physical or mental balance. A stressful event, such as a layoff, divorce, or tragic life event, can trigger our fight-or-flight response. This can cause hormones like adrenaline to surge throughout our bodies.

There is also "acute stress," which is less extreme, but also releases adrenaline in the body; acute stress is exciting. This is the rush of going skydiving, the spark of chemistry that ignites when you meet someone new that could be the one, the thrill of walking onstage for your first presentation at the start of your new speaking career. Stress keeps us alive and active.

Stress itself is something many of us relate to, but most of us, whether we realize it or not, are actually addicted to stress. Stress helps us feel important, needed, busy, and alive. Because adrenaline and cortisol are released in our bodies when we feel stressed, stress causes us to relate to the world with a heightened sense of awareness.

When I started my own business, stress was my middle name. I was always so busy. Friends were getting married, having baby showers, having babies, and I constantly found myself saying that I was too busy and stressed out to show up to plan parties or to join the decoration committee. I would show up for the actual events, but I was always so overwhelmed. I remember always thinking, "I can't stay long because I have to get back to work." It wasn't until one year after my best friend's baby was born that I finally found an opening in my ridiculously "busy" life to babysit for her little fella. I was on the floor playing with her cute little guy, and I had an epiphany; I realized my fallback to stress was actually keeping me from living my life fully. I was so busy trying to create a future life that I was actually missing my current life. I had a brand and blog called Play with the World, but my best friend had a child for an entire year, and yet this was the first time I was spending quality time with him. This moment helped me go deep into my own attachment to the notorious emotion I identified with, the lovely stress. And I finally realized that the amount of stress I felt was in direct proportion to the lack of control I felt. I was building a business and worried about if it would be a success. In order to control the outcome, I channeled all my energy into work. I was focusing my attention on something I felt was important, but I was doing it to an extreme. I was giving it too much focus, and shortchanging everything else in my life. Although I enjoyed my work, it had become my entire life. I didn't have any weekends, and my time off was always spent brainstorming work ideas. My attention was focused on building a successful business, but I gave up the time I needed to play. I sacrificed my true needs to connect with friends and family in an effort to make my business success-ful. Because I didn't trust how my business would turn out, I channeled everything I had into it and gave up my life. This caused intense stress because I was ignoring and avoiding my true needs. We often feel stress because we are overworking or over-worrying in an area of our life. The stress creeps in to remind us that we are actually out of balance.

Although I was stressed out, it was a different type of stress than my best friend had. She too had spent that past year in a constant state of stress, raising a first newborn baby, adapting to a new lifestyle, focusing all of her energy on raising and protecting this little sweet fella, so that everything else in her life fell by the wayside. Her workout schedules all but vanished, she stopped calling me just to chat and catch up, and her attention and stress was all tied to this beautiful new boy. This is the type of stress that invigorates us. But it is stress nonetheless, and the key is knowing how to deal with it.

How we deal with stress and attach it to the events in our life is the connection that can lead us to happiness. Stress can actually help us through difficult and challenging times. We let stress become the main focus of our life in order to power through things we seemingly might not get through otherwise. Stress is the power that helps us adapt to new situations in life. On any given day, **the amount of stress we all feel is in direct proportion to how out of control we feel.** We hold on to stress because it gives us a sense of control. We want to control our environment and we hope to cre-ate predictable circumstances. This is why we work so hard to grow our own new business or protect our newborn children. We try to make things happen. So in knowing that stress is part of life, what if our attachment to stress isn't the problem; what if the problem is how we look at stress?

In the 2013 TED Talk "How to Make Stress Your Friend,"

health psychologist Kelly McGonigal reveals a fascinating new concept that the harmful effects of stress may be a consequence of our perception that it is bad for our health. "Can changing how you think about stress make you healthier? Here the science says yes," says McGonigal. "Your heart might be pounding, you may be breathing faster . . . but what if you viewed them as signs that your body was energized and it's preparing you to meet this challenge." The TED blog post (blog.ted.com/could-stress-be-good-for-you-recent-research-that-suggests-it-has-benefits/) on this topic goes deeper. The post reiterates that stress may actually be connected to longevity—if a person doesn't view it as a negative. Researchers polled almost 29,000 people, asking them to rate their level of stress over the previous year, as well as how much they believed this stress influenced their health. The researchers looked at public death records over the next eight years to see if any subjects had passed away. They found that there findings were correct: People who reported having high levels of stress and who believed stress had a large impact on their health had a 43 percent increased risk of death. On the other hand, those that experienced a lot of stress but did not perceive its effects as negative were less likely to die.

What this research suggests is that stress is only bad if we think it's bad.

When we change our perceptions of "bad" or "stressful" things we can change their effect on us. As the research states, if the person doesn't view stress as negative it won't affect them as much. This is a brave new concept that I applied to my own life when it came to stress around my addictions. The concept worked so well I started using it in my coaching practice, and clients all around the world have seen great results. Many people come to me wanting to break addictions, just like I once did. Although Kelly McGonigal was talking about addiction to stress, I applied this same principle to my own life with other areas where I had a negative perception or addiction, and I saw a healing transformation. One thing that helped me heal my food addiction was shifting my "stress" and "shame" around the addiction. By removing the "negative perception" around it, the addiction itself had less of a hold and I was able to focus on healing the patterns and find a healthier alternative.

Many of us have unhealthy behaviors that stress us out immensely. We punish ourselves for being addicted to substances or things that are not good for us. We become our own personal punching bag as we shame and mentally abuse ourselves.

This radical new wave of research suggests that how you feel about patterns, habits, or situations in your life is more important than the actual habit itself, which I found to be true in my own life.

When I held on to the belief that I was bad for overeating, it would grow in my mind like a monster under the bed. The shadows would override any ounce of hope and healing. The darkness of guilt would make me feel horrible, and my addiction cycle would continue. It wasn't until I applied the Kelly McGonigal approach to letting go of the stress to the stress I felt about my food addictions that the habits lifted. My food addictions became less dramatic, the guilt disappeared, and my stress levels balanced out. Instead of saying to myself, "That ice cream and chocolate cake are bad, and I am a horrible person for eating all that sugar!" I switched to a more compassionate, less stressed-out approach: "Ice cream sounds pretty good right now. I am thankful for these glorious flavors. I am celebrating life by enjoying this wonderful treat." I removed the stress and negativity around eating and food being "bad," and my food addiction lifted. I turned my judgment into compassion, and I started to eat less, and lost weight. My food addiction was in part cured because I released the stress around the habit. I'm not diminishing the harmfulness of addictions and therapies needed to help individuals overcome them. All

I am suggesting is we take away the emotional pain and burdensome stress tied to our habits so the healing can occur. How we think about what we do is just as important as what we actually do. Turning off the negative critic will help the healing happen faster.

When we stop hating ourselves because of our problems and show ourselves self-love, we can work on helping ourselves overcome them with more grace and ease. I, as well as many coaching clients, have had powerful breakthroughs by trying this approach; when we can remove the self-blame from our habits, and adopt a more compassionate self-loving approach, we feel more happy and peaceful. Now it is your turn to try it out.

∽

JOY ROUTE
Let go.

The joy route to releasing this habit hindering our happiness is to access our inner joy. We do this by letting go. This joy route concept is derived from my own personal exploration of healing my own addictions.

Many years ago I was suffering from multiple eating disorders. I was bulimic and a food addict. This caused me enormous amounts of stress, as I would fight with myself, always wondering why I was so damaged. Being the victim of an addiction or disorder can cause enormous amounts of self-sabotage if we don't check ourselves. Most of us walk around feeling wounded, damaged, and guilty, when the bottom line is we really just want to enjoy the things we resist. For me, my food addictions and out-of-control binge-fests were a result of denying who I really was. I was ignoring my authentic self, my true self, the person who LOVES food. I was avoiding my joy route. The real me wanted to try new foods and taste the flavors and smell the aromas, but sometimes "eating" certain types of food when you are overweight is considered a social stigma. I stayed addicted to food and overate because of this stigma, which caused enormous amounts of stress in my life. It wasn't until I let go of the notion that my "addiction" and habits were "bad" that my world transformed. Over time, slowly my disorders lifted and my experience with food shifted. I started to appreciate my food; I was present with it and I chose to enjoy each bite fully. By doing this, my attachment to needing more lifted. I was no longer stressed out about my meals. My thoughts no longer circled around what I was going to eat or when I would eat, and the attachment lessened its hold on me. Because I wasn't so stressed out about it, I was able to get to the root cause. I did this by letting go of thinking it was bad. I did this by following my joy route.

You see, all of us have an inner desire to connect with the things we gravitate toward. Most attachments, habits, and patterns that cause us stress are actually in our life because they are helping us in an indirect way. If we didn't have the attachment or stress, it would cause more havoc for us. Looking at your attachments as a process can help you remove stress around those habits. The key here is to remove the stress. Because addictions and attachments cause real chemical changes in the body, withdrawal is very real and often painful, whether it is cocaine, alcohol, sugar, or sex. When we are attached or addicted to anything, it is always a layered process to heal. But removing the stress and personal pressure we put on ourselves is one small step that can transform the patterns in a grand way.

Let's put it into action.

Think about your own life and a habit you have been trying to quit. Is there stress around this habit because you, or society, believe it is "bad"? Here is how we can break up with our habit of being attached to things that cause us stress.

AWESOME ACTION 1: Identify Your Habit or Attachment and Your Current Beliefs About It

What habit or attachment is causing you the most stress in your life right now?

AWESOME ACTION 2: Turn Your Bad into Glad

Instead of looking at your habit or attachment as bad, turn it into a learning experience. Be glad for the situation because it is helping you learn more about yourself. Ask yourself what you can learn from this attachment.

To access more joy, and to release the emotional hold of your habit or addiction, repeat this motivational mantra:

> "My problems are not actually problems or barriers, they are pathways."

AWESOME ACTION 3: Create a Let Go List

A Let Go List has saved me multiple times on my journey to self-love and happiness. A Let Go List is kind of like a gratitude list, but instead of listing out what you are thankful for, you list what you want to let go of. I refer to my Let Go List daily. This has helped me maintain a recovered life free of drugs and depression. I also do this at the start of every New Year and the results are powerful. Your list could include people, habits, beliefs, or situations you want to release. A Let Go List is something to carry with you when you are feeling stuck or stressed out.

It could be as simple as asking yourself, "What is no longer serving me? What do I need to let go of today?" This is what I ask myself daily, and it helps me maintain balance and an attachment-free life. Our stress, remember, is caused by feeling out of control, and because we want certainty, we create stress to give us a sense of control. To create your Let Go List, ask yourself how much stress you are carrying around. Do you feel burdened by life's circumstances and emotional issues? Becoming more grounded and happy starts with letting go of worry and stress.

As I said, I learned this in my own journey. In the process, I had to let go of a lot of things to become the person I am today. The Let Go List comes in handy when you want to become a healthier version of who you are today. If you are stuck in a depression, or feel trapped in an addiction, it may feel like the world is caving in on you. You can pull out of this emotional state by going deeper inward and releasing what no longer serves you. You do this in the Let Go List.

Physically, spiritually, and emotionally, I had to learn how to let go of the person I thought I should be in order to be the person I really wanted to be. Letting go of anything in life can be a little scary, but it can also be an amazing act of self-love.

Letting go of your worries and stress will make a difference for your future. Trust me, your future self will thank you, and you will find that the stresses you feel for these situations will disappear in the process. Take time to create a list for yourself. What are you ready to let go of?

I created a go-to list of things you might want to let go of. Create your own list, but you can use this one to get you started. I published this list on my site playwiththeworld.com, and it has been shared across social media channels almost one million times. The reason I think this list resonates with so many is because we all have "stuff" we want to let go of. Please allow this list to help.

Twenty Things to Let Go of in Order to Reach Unlimited Happiness

1. Let go of all thoughts that don't make you feel empowered and strong.
2. Let go of feeling guilty for doing what you truly want to do.
3. Let go of the fear of the unknown; take one small step and watch the path reveal itself.
4. Let go of regrets; at one point in your life, that "whatever" was exactly what you wanted and needed.
5. Let go of worrying; worrying is like praying to receive what you don't want.
6. Let go of blaming anyone for anything; be accountable for your own life. If you don't like something, you have two choices: Accept it or change it.
7. Let go of thinking you are damaged; you matter, and the world needs you just as you are.
8. Let go of thinking your dreams are not important; always follow your heart.
9. Let go of being the "go-to person" for everyone, all the time; stop blowing yourself off and take care of you first . . . because you matter.
10. Let go of thinking everyone else is happier, more successful, or better off than you. You are right where you need to be. Your journey is unfolding perfectly for you.
11. Let go of thinking there's a right and wrong way to do things or to see the world. Enjoy the contrast and celebrate the diversity and richness of life.
12. Let go of cheating on your future with your past. It's time to move on and tell a new story.
13. Let go of thinking you are not where you should be. You are

right where you need to be to get to where you want to go, so start asking yourself where you want to go.

14. Let go of anger toward ex-lovers and family. We all deserve happiness and love; just because it is over doesn't mean the love was wrong.

15. Let go of the need to do more and be more; for today, you've done the best you can and that is enough.

16. Let go of thinking you have to know how to make it happen; we learn the way on the way.

17. Let go of your money woes; make a plan to pay off debt and focus on your abundance.

18. Let go of trying to save or change people. Everyone has their own path, and the best thing you can do is work on yourself and stop focusing on others.

19. Let go of trying to fit in and be accepted by everyone. Your uniqueness is what makes you outstanding.

20. Let go of self-hate. You are not the shape of your body or the number on the scale. Who you are matters, and the world needs you as you are. Celebrate you!

~ↄ

MOTIVATIONAL MANTRAS

"I am perfect as I am.
I allow myself to be who I really want to be.
It is safe to show my true self."

TWENTY-ONE

Play with the World

❧

HABIT HINDERING HAPPINESS
We think happiness is outside ourselves.

We can be in only one of two states: Either the mind is running us or we are running our mind. Yes, we know that happiness is a choice, but sometimes choosing happy can be hard. This is because for so many of us, in the pursuit of happiness we listen to our mind running rampant. At this stage of our journey together, you probably can see that lasting happiness is dependent on how much we can quit the mind. When we are in tune with our body and our mind and in touch with our heart's desires, we can feel genuine happiness.

Today, I consider myself an extremely happy person, but it hasn't always been that way. The truth is that I've made HUGE strides to be where I am today. I had to dig deep inside myself to access authentic joy, the kind that cannot be manufactured by false promises and one-night-stand mantras spit out by pop psychologists. If you still fall into depression or if life doesn't make sense right now, you're not alone. We all have moments of frustration. Resisting these feelings actually keeps us from being happy.

I work with a lot of clients who are on a spiritual path, and they tell me they feel bad for being angry, or they feel like the spiritual thing to do is to not get jealous. The reality is, we are humans walking around on earth having human experiences. I believe we are spiritual beings having a human experience instead of being humans striving for a spiritual experience. This means that we try so hard to be happy, or feel enlightenment, or reach joy that it actually prevents us from reaching it, because we are not designed to be in utopia 24/7. Yes, happiness is a choice and you can certainly choose to feel joy in every moment, but know that life happens, human experiences rush in to remind us we are on earth fumbling, trying, working through stuff to overcome and rise above. Be compassionate with yourself and embrace your humanity.

So many of my coaching clients first come to me and tell me they don't know how to be happy, they feel numb inside, and they always feel like they are searching for something but can't find it, nor do they know what it is. I know this feeling too well; I spent over twenty years of my life suffering through this pain. The actions in this book certainly help to recondition ourselves to focus on what we really want, but after this book is read and the laptop or electronic devices are closed down, it is the practice that counts. Putting happiness into our life is about a dedicated practice. Just like working out or mastering a new skill, we must allow ourselves to be beginners at first. Many of us stumble and get mad at ourselves because we feel like we aren't getting happy; this only adds intense pressure that prevents us from moving forward. When my clients express their guilt, fear, or shame, I work with them to embrace it. At first it is a very foreign concept and they are confused, shocked, and a little worried; they look at me like I'm nuts. But every time they do go into the emotion and embrace the anger, resentment, jealousy, shame, or guilt, they come out with fewer bruises, and more awareness and inner peace. The thing about emotions is they are part of being human. So stop saying to yourself, "I shouldn't feel this way, this is not what happy people do, or how spiritual people feel." You are actually hurting yourself; you are trying to convince yourself that you need to be different from what you really are yearning to express in that moment.

Recently, I shared this method with a new client whom I was coaching via Skype. He had so much inner turmoil and stress. He was feeling very confused by his life and couldn't understand why he couldn't be happy. He had a great supportive girlfriend, a decent job, but he just felt disconnected from everything. He expressed that he was carrying around a lot of self-pity, guilt, and shame. He asked me, "Why is it so hard to be happy?" I compassionately said, "Because you are TRYING to be happy." His eyes lit up and he seemed to understand. He said, "Yes I am trying because I want to be happy, but I see what you are saying because I am trying, I am focusing on how I am not happy." BINGO! The happiest people in the world don't try, they just are and they honor where they are in each moment, and let the emotions they are feeling pass through them rather than resisting and holding on to them. I asked my client, "When is the last time you really felt genuinely happy?" He thought for a moment and smiled with a goofy childlike grin and said, "When I played the bongo drums, but it has been years." I told him his awesome opportunity this week was to play the drums. He froze up and said, "Oh man, but it has been so long." I asked, "Where are your bongos?" He told me they were in his closet and I encouraged him to pull them out and play something for me. He reluctantly obliged and performed a mini–jam session. Almost immediately I saw a light ignite within him. He gave himself time to be. He chose happy. He chose to act on the inspiration that was pulling him, he chose to do what he loves. And when he did, he connected to his happiness. In our next session, he told me he was doing much better, he met up with his buddies for a full-out jam session, and he now schedules his happiness habit into his weekly and daily routine. Scheduling happiness is important for maintaining a happy life. Instead of spending all of our time on how we are not happy, or chasing happiness outside of ourselves, we do things that make us happy. The more things we do that bring us joy, the happier and more fulfilled we will be.

When I was in corporate suffocating with depression, I never made joy a priority. I simply went through the motions at work and returned home to stuff my face with high-calorie food, then threw it up in the toilet. Today, as I write this chapter, my life is much different. I live in my favorite place in the world, Hawaii; I woke up this morning with a smile on my face; I said thank you to the universe for a another opportunity to live a full day; and I said I love you in the mirror as I brushed my teeth. I put my swimsuit on and went surfing for two hours. I connected with locals and smiled at strangers. I went to my favorite health food café on the island, and right now I am sitting here drinking fresh green juice and fueling up with a healthy acai bowl. I am passionate about my job, which actually doesn't feel like a job at all. My life is very different than it was several years ago.

It all comes down to respect. We have to respect ourselves enough to believe we are worth lasting happiness. Respecting yourself doesn't have to start tomorrow after your addictions are healed or after you reach a happy place. Respect starts right now, in this moment. When you reach for happiness, the joy you have access to—your drum set, your surfboard, your feel-good healthy food— these mini-moments pile up to create an extraordinary life. I didn't just wake up one day and say I respect myself and now I am happy. It was daily action, small mini-steps. But choosing to follow my joy was the essential ingredient. Give yourself permission to do what makes you happy. Follow your heart's pull. Play your drums, dance your beat, surf your wave. When we deny ourselves life, we suffocate happiness. Choose your life. Living it fully starts with one step at a time. Take that step. Play with the world.

∽

JOY ROUTE
Play with the world.

I started the website playwiththeworld.com to help shine light in the darkness. It is a result of me following my heart and creating a space online where people can come and have a retreat for their soul. Play With The World is not about travel or adventure (although I am a travel writer and adventure buff); it is about taking that step and moving toward happiness. For me it is traveling and playing in nature and having new adventures. But I know that not everyone is obsessed with travel or in love with adrenaline-fueled activities. But I do know that everyone is craving happiness. Even when we are happy, we want to stay happy. So Play With the World is the joy route to cure our anxieties and self-sabotaging habits. When we play, which means we take steps to follow through on what brings us joy, we are uplifted, inspired, and connected to our best self. Just like my client who gave himself permission to play his bongos: He stopped talking and thinking about how he was unhappy and he took action and just did it; he played the drums. So push play on your joy route and access your own inspiration. Play With the World is all about playing with your world despite the conditions of the world. You can still be happy when things are going bad. You can still be happy if you don't have a lot of money or as much as you think you need. You can still be happy if you aren't in your dream job or with your soul mate. You can still be happy IN THIS MOMENT, RIGHT NOW by playing with the world around you and being fully present for the experience. When I was depressed and struggling with eating disorders and a terrible body image, I tried this method out and it saved my life. My issues dropped away, the clarity came rushing in, and I chose happiness and hope.

I save every email I get from clients and readers who reconnect with their joy. Artists sending me illustrations, musicians telling me they got back into the studio, aspiring authors telling me they found their happy by putting pen to paper. Do it, just do it! My heart is so full of love when I do what I love, and I want the same thing for you. You know what you love. You don't have to find it. Just go back to when you felt it. When were you fully engaged and in love? We are all born with certain things that bring us joy, but we grow up and lose sight of them. So the best thing to do is grow up and be a kid again.

I was just invited to be a presenter in Mexico at Las Olas Surf Safaris where their motto is "We make girls out of women." Such a perfect collaboration, because playing with the world is all about getting back to the joy of life and feeling the expansiveness, the joy-filled moments that come with being a child. Think about it: Children are curious, excited for life, eager to try new things, and are usually present in the moment, especially when it is something they love to do. My mother always tells me I was so easy growing up because she just set up an art table in the yard and I would paint, draw, and write for hours and hours. I was so happy and connected to myself when I expressed myself creatively and when I was in nature. I would write poetry in the grass while other children ran around playing tag.

Doing what you love and connecting with your true self is what Play With The World is all about. You can stop searching for happiness when you recognize the happiness already inside of you.

Play with the World 291

AWESOME ACTION 1: Play with the World

Okay, friends, you have worked so hard and done so much amazing work. This has been an intense process, but you are now in a position to live your full potential so the only awesome action here is to Go PLAY WITH THE WORLD.

You know what to do. Everything you need is inside of you. Now it is time to take real action. Play, have fun, choose joy, respect yourself to know that you deserve the very best. You, my friend, are ready to fly. Go be your amazing self and have a blast playing with the world.

MOTIVATIONAL MANTRA

This chapter's motivational mantra is different. Instead of giving you one power line, I've chosen to leave you with this go-to list for lasting happiness. If ever on your journey you feel stuck or out of alignment lean on this list. Whenever I feel out of alignment, I return to this list and it gets me back on track.

TWENTY-FIVE ADVENTURES FOR YOUR SOUL TO KEEP YOUR HAPPY

1. Stop worrying; if it is supposed to happen it will.
2. Allow yourself to be a beginner. No one starts off being excellent.
3. Don't let your happiness depend on anything outside yourself.
4. Stay close to everything that makes you feel alive.
5. Listen to your body; it will lead you to unlimited health.
6. Surround yourself with people who see your greatness.
7. Make peace with your past.

8. See all setbacks as growth opportunities.
9. Comparing yourself to others will hurt your health and steal your joy.
10. Don't give up, EVER. You are closer than you think to realizing your goal.
11. You always have a choice.
12. Stop chasing what's not working.
13. Believe wholeheartedly in miracles.
14. Don't postpone joy.
15. Trust the universe; there is a plan greater than yours.
16. Wake up every morning with a grateful heart.
17. Remember things take time.
18. Always trust your gut.
19. No need to change people; just love them for who they are.
20. Don't resist change.
21. Forgive yourself.
22. Your life is a creative adventure.
23. Release expectations and enjoy the journey; there is no destination.
24. Just do you.
25. You're not broken or damaged. You are perfect just the way you are.

The End

But really, it's just the beginning for you and your new awesome passion-filled life.

The End

Afterword

When I first created the proposal for this book, I assumed my adventure would be all weight loss. When I lost the extra body weight, I would be able to be comfortable in my skin. What I didn't expect was the real gift this book gave me: the gift of self-acceptance.

So many of us spend precious moments consumed with self-hate, worry, and anxiety. We spend enormous amounts of time, energy, and money trying to be someone else, somewhere else, or resisting where and who we really are. Acceptance is about releasing resistance. Acceptance is the key to a happy life.

I've been in Hawaii for almost three months now, and I made a promise to myself that while writing this book I would not get on a scale. Now that it is done, I decided yesterday I was allowed to check my weight, and to my surprise I gained five pounds. The surprise is not that I gained weight, but my reaction to it. For the first time in my life, I was comfortable. I said to myself, "I am happier than I have ever been. I am more comfortable in my body than I have ever been, and I am more in love with myself and life than I ever thought possible." The reality is, I gained so much more than what I thought I would lose.

So there you have it. It was never about the number on the scale. It was about learning how to be alive in my life, to fully be present, and respect and honor this body. Fully accepting myself means showing up for myself and consciously choosing joy. **The more joy we feel, the less struggle we face.**

Sometimes we set out on a mission to get happy and we think we will get what we want, but you can rest assured the universe will swoop in and give you what you really need.

Adventures for Your Soul is about you stepping fully into your own life and embracing yourself completely. It is about respecting yourself enough to know that your dreams, your goals, and your path matter.

As I write this final section, I am poolside at the Ritz-Carlton in Maui, Hawaii. I led a virtual corporate workshop this morning for women living in Cincinnati. I could have led the workshop from the place I am renting, but I didn't want to settle. I choose to show up fully for the workshop participants and for myself. I didn't have to check myself into one of the fanciest resorts on the island; I didn't have to, I chose to.

Living on purpose means we make choices that align with our values. I choose to put myself into my own life and not settle. Do not settle. Your life is too precious to spend any more time on earth doing anything that does not make your soul sing. Respect yourself enough to know that you deserve the absolute very best.

Full acceptance of who you are and why you are here is the greatest gift of all. *Adventures for Your Soul* is not about changing you, or fixing mistakes, or reversing what is broken. This process is about allowing yourself to be who you really are, free of self-criticism, emotional strain, and inner turmoil. Because life is much easier when we are not at war with ourselves. Becoming your own best friend is a gift only you can give yourself. It is not about becoming anything, or changing anything about us, but rather letting the real you shine through; it comes back to embracing who we really are.

Maybe the journey of life isn't so much about becoming any one thing or accomplishing any one goal. We spend so much time trying to get "there" and be someone we think we need to be, but what if it is about *un-becoming* every single thing that isn't really true to you so you can be who you were really meant to be in the first place?

And so it is. You belong just as you are. You matter.

Acknowledgments

This book has been a dream in my heart for many years. I am so thankful it has made it into the world and with the vision and support of so many wonderful people. I am thankful for all of the support, love, and friendship along the way.

Tremendous hugs to my family, my best friends, and support system: Dad, Mom, Clint, Rhonda, Aunt Linda, and Heidi. You're the best. You each support my every crazy move in life and are always there with patience, kind words, and love. You each make it possible for me to spread my wings.

Marita, your friendship since I first met you in Brazil has helped me grow into my dreams and realize my potential. You are such a beautiful person. I love you, soul sister!

My dear author friends: Gabrielle Bernstein, Christine Arylo, Kristine Carlson, Amy Ahlers, Christine Hassler, Rhonda Britten, Amy Leigh Mercree, Karen Salmansohn, and Katrina Love Sean. Thank you for your guidance, love, and support for this work. And thank you, *MindBodyGreen* editors, for supporting my writing career and helping me spread the message of hope and happiness to the masses.

My gurus, mentors, and teachers, Summer Bacon, James Martin Peebles, John of God, Esther Hicks and the Abrahams, my Angels, and of course God, I am thankful for your constant nudges and support in writing this book.

A huge heartfelt hug and thanks to my amazing literary agents at MDM Management, Gabriel, Steve, and Michelle. To the amazing support system at the Berkley Publishing Group, thank you for believing and seeing the potential in this work and helping me share it with the world. Denise, you're an amazing person to work with. Thank you for believing in this message and helping me get it out into the world.

Thank you, dear reader and the PlayWiththeWorld.com community. I wake up every day so excited to do what I do—for you. You inspire me to keep going with your messages, support, and enthusiasm for this work.

And last but not least, Tucker, you are my hero. You came to me at the darkest period of my life and pulled me into the light. You are the best buddy I could ever ask for and the coolest golden retriever in the world. Thanks for finding me. I love you. For all of the remarkable encounters and folks I've met over the years, I am deeply grateful and forever blessed.

About the Author

Shannon Kaiser has been labeled among the Top 100 Women to Watch in Wellness by *MindBodyGreen*, and a modern thought leader on the rise by CaféTruth. She is the bestselling author of *Find Your Happy: An Inspirational Guide to Loving Life to Its Fullest*, and a six-time contributing author to *Chicken Soup for the Soul*. She is an inspirational author, speaker, travel writer, and international life coach who left her successful career in advertising several years ago to follow her heart and be a writer. Her unique and adventurous twist to self-help inspires people to take risks and embrace the unknown so they can live openly and courageously from their heart.

Her website PlayWithTheWorld.com was named one of the Top 100 Self-Help Blogs and Top 75 Personal Growth websites on the Internet by the Institute for the Psychology of Eating.

Her sought-after ideas have been featured in media outlets across the world such as *Good Morning America*, *Good Day New York*, *Inside Edition*, *Health* Magazine, *Women's Health*, *Conde Nast Traveler*, and HuffPost Live, and she is a regular contributor

for *The Huffington Post*, *MindBodyGreen*, *Healing Lifestyles &
Spas*, Examiner.com, Tiny Buddha, and The Daily Love. When
she isn't travel writing, she lives in Portland, Oregon, with her
adventure buddy, her dog, Tucker.

For coaching sessions and inquires contact
coach@playwiththeworld.com.

For more information about Shannon Kaiser and her signature
Play With The World approach to life and breakthrough
transformational workshops, lectures, and events please visit:
www.playwiththeworld.com.